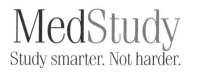

MedStudy
Study smarter. Not harder.

Pediatrics
Answers to Board-Style Questions

Q&A 1

Edited by J. Thomas Cross, Jr., MD, MPH

NOTICE: These Question and Answer books are intended as a supplementary study tool for the Pediatric Certification and Recertification exams. These books are an excellent self study and self-assessment tool in preparing for the ABP exams in conjunction with your favorite textbook of Pediatrics. MedStudy will publish a Core Curriculum for Pediatrics in the Fall of 2003.

GOOD STUDYING!

This material is authored by J. Thomas Cross, Jr., MD, MPH
Publisher: MedStudy Corporation

MEDSTUDY CORPORATION
800-841-0547

1. Answer: A

The correct answer is that her son has the developmental age of approximately 4 months. A 7-month old infant should be able to do the following things: lift their head, roll over and crawl or creep-crawl, sit briefly with the support of pelvis, when held erect they should support most of their weight and actively bounce. They should reach out and grasp objects and be able to transfer them from hand to hand, and they should babble and respond to changes in the emotional content of a social contact. Ms. Andrews' infant has the developmental age of approximately 4 months. Ms. Andrews was correct in her assessment of the situation and an evaluation of the infant should begin to attempt to identify reasons for the significant developmental delay this infant has.

2. Answer: C

The correct answer is her infant has normal developmental milestones for an 8-week-old. An 8-week-old should be able to do all those developmental tasks outlined in the physical examination above. A 4-week-old can only momentarily raise their head to the plane of the body on ventral suspension. The head lag is normal to both a 4 and 8-week-old infant, while a 4-week old will watch an object move, they will not watch it for 180°. A 4-week old is only beginning to smile and moves their body in cadence with the voice of others in a social situation. A newborn cannot support their head, has a predominance of primitive reflexes present (e.g., Moro, palmar and plantar grasps) and has a visual preference for the human face.

3. Answer: D

The correct answer is her son has a developmental age of a 9-month-old. By one year of age a child should be able to rise independently and take several steps without assistance. Children usually start walking with one hand held by 11 months of age. By their first birthday a child should not only pick up an object using a pincer grasp but should release the object to another person upon request or gesture. They should know a few words besides mama or dada and they should be able to play a simple ball game. Although the history of meningitis might be the cause of his delay it is important to note that dad also has had some learning difficulties in his life and more information would be needed to make sure there are no other factors contributing to the developmental delay in this child. It would be too early to say what type of classes this child would be able to attend by the time he was of middle school age.

4. Answer: B

The correct answer is that she has the developmental age of a 15 month old. An 18-month-old should be able to run stiffly, sit on a small chair, and walk up stairs with one hand held. They should make a tower of 4 cubes and imitate scribbling as well as dump a pellet from the bottle. They should use about 10 words on average and be able to identify one or more body parts. They should feed themselves and seek help when in trouble. A 24-month-old should run well and be able to walk up and down the stairs one step at a time. They should be able to make a tower of 7 cubes and make circular scribbling. They should be able to put three words together (e.g., subject, verb, object) and tell others of their immediate experiences. A 30-month-old goes up and down the stairs alternating their feet, makes a tower of 9 cubes, refers to self as "I", and will know their full name. Although the history of the labor and delivery is suggestive of potential birth problems there is insufficient data to prove this and other etiologies of developmental delay should be sought.

5. Answer: A

The correct answer is that based upon her weight, height, head circumference and her developmental examination, she is approximately 18 months of age. The average weight, height, and head circumference for a 12-month old girl is approximately 10 kg, 75 cm, and 45 cm. For a 24 month old girl the average weight, height and head circumference is approximately 12 kg, 86 cm, and 48 cm, so reviewing growth curves, her anthropometric values would place her between 12 and 24 months of age. Based upon her developmental examination she does everything an 18 month-old infant should do. A 12-month–old can walk on level ground with one hand held but not steps, can pick up a pellet with a pincer grasp but not place it in a bottle, and might only say a few words (besides mama, dada). A 15-month-old should walk alone but crawl up stairs, make a tower of 3 cubes and be able to insert a pellet into a bottle, follow simple commands, just start speaking their first real words, and indicate some desires by pointing. A 24 month old should run well, walk up and down stairs one step at a time, make a tower of 7 cubes, put three words together, and should handle a spoon well.

6. Answer: E

The correct answer is that Adam's development is appropriate for his age. He is more advanced than a 24-month-old child who should be able to run well and walk up and down the stairs one step at a time, but a 24-month-old should not be able to stand on one foot. A 24-month-old should only be able to stack 7 cubes and can only imitate horizontal strokes. A 24-month-old should only be able to put 3 words together. Adam is not as advanced as a 48-month-old child. A 48-month-old child should be able to hop on one foot instead of standing momentarily on one foot. They should also be able to copy a cross and a square instead of a circle. Besides being able to dress themselves they should be able to go to the toilet alone. The choice of what type of school classes he will be able to attend will be decided upon school entry. There is no reason to remove him from day care.

7. Answer: C

The correct answer is Michael has the appropriate developmental skills to attend kindergarten. Michael is doing the items that are appropriate for a child of 5 years of age. A 2-year-old should be able to run, a three-year-old should ride a tricycle, a four-year-old should be able to hop on one foot and a 5-year-old should be able to skip. An 18-month-old should imitate a vertical line and a 24-month-old should imitate a horizontal line. A 30-month-old will make both a vertical and a horizontal stoke but will not join them to make a cross. A 3-year-old will copy a cross, a 4-year-old will copy a cross and a square and a 5-year-old will copy a triangle. A 3-year-old will start helping to dressing themselves and by the time they are five they can dress and undress themselves. A 4-year-old can count 4 pennies accurately and a 5-year-old can count 10 pennies. A five-year-old should know 4 colors.

8. Answer: A

The correct answer is walk independently. Most 9 month olds can do most of these things except walk independently. Occasionally you will see a 9 month old who can walk, but it certainly is of no concern if he doesn't. Usually by 12-15 months, most children can walk.

9. Answer: B

The correct answer is use 2 or 3 word sentences. Most children do not begin using 2 or 3 word sentences until they are 24 months old. All of the other answers are typical of 18 month olds.

10. Answer: C

The correct answer is reassure mother that attacks are harmless and will eventually resolve on their own. This scenario is very typical of breath-holding spells. Peak age of onset is 6 months to 2 years of age. After the child passes out, they can become rigid and one-third can progress to muscle twitches which often makes the parents think it is a seizure. They resume normal breathing and become fully alert within 1 minute. An EEG is only necessary if the spell is atypical or lasts longer than 1 minute. Refer to a cardiologist if it is a pallid spell. Electrolytes will be normal and are unnecessary. It is very scary for parents, but reassure the mother that her child will be fine. Tell her to have the child lie down during the attack. After the attack, she can give the child a brief hug but then go about her business. If the spell was caused because the child did not get her way, do not give in to her after the attack because it may cause deliberate breath-holding spells.

11. Answer: B

The correct "incorrect" answer is soiling accidents are the responsibility of both the child and the parent and they equally should be involved in the clean-up. Soiling accidents should be the responsibility of the child with parents rendering a MINIMAL level of assistance depending on the age and developmental level of the child. Whenever, a parent detects soiling, the child needs to clean up and change clothing on the first request. In exchange for this level of cooperation, it is understood that the child will not receive any punishment or admonitions from the parent. It is recommended that the child sit on the toilet, preferably 2 times a day, for intervals of 5 to 10 minutes. Some children are resistant to sitting due to fear of having painful bowel movements and this should be alleviated by the use of non-stimulant stool softeners. Refusal to sit on the toilet should always be met with a privilege restriction.

12. Answer: D

The correct "incorrect" answer is use of a "potty-alarm" is appropriate for children aged 4 years and above. These are quite effective, approaching 80% initial success rates, but are only useful in children at least 6 to 7 years of age. The other items are true. "Overcorrection" is a technique whereby parents tell the child to return to the bathroom 5 minutes after voiding to "try again" and then return in another 5 minutes. Usually the child will void a small amount of residual urine on one of the return trips. This is useful if the child has a habit of not emptying their bladder completely during voiding and thus leak urine for a period of time after—leaving them with damp but not soaked underwear. Reward systems are useful in all treatments for enuresis as well as encopresis.

13. Answer: A

The correct answer is pica is frequently associated with mental retardation. Most cases usually begin to occur between 12 and 18 months. It can lead to medical complications such as lead poisoning, nutritional deficiencies, and obstruction. In the case of potentially dangerous pica, use of mild punishment is sometimes recommended. Dangerous items should always be removed quickly from a child and the child should never be allowed to dispose of such items. It is best to praise a child if they have appropriately avoided putting a potential pica agent in their mouth.

14. Answer: E

The correct answer is the child needs to be quiet and physically in control by the end of the time-out or it is extended. Time out is NOT instinctive for children—they must be taught how to take a time-out. A warning that a time-out is coming will only prolong the temper tantrum. Time-outs do not lose their usefulness when a child says that they do not mind or even like time-outs—it is supposed to reduce inappropriate behavior over time and it not supposed to be a "miserable" experience. After a time-out, short term restitution is ok (like picking up the toys they threw), but thereafter it is best to provide positive reinforcement for good behavior.

15. Answer: C

The correct answer is enormous growth in the number and branching of dendrites and the multiplication of complex synaptic junctions occurs. The brain quadruples in size from 350g in the newborn to 1450 grams in the adult.

16. Answer: D

The correct answer is the amount of enrichment of adult-infant social interactions. Infants who are raised in institutions staffed by few and inconsistent caretakers display marked retardation in adaptive behavior. Rapid and complete recovery can occur if adoption into family life occurs before the end of the first year.

17. Answer: A

The correct answer is magical thinking. Children from 2 to 7 years of age are in the preoperational stage of development. This period generally is presented in two manners---1) immanent justice—the child perceives their own illness as a punishment for some misdeed or 2) magical thinking—referring to the belief that they can wish the disease away. Concrete operations do not occur generally until 7 to 11 years of age and formal operations will not appear until 12 to 18 years of age. Peer acceptance would be a concern for the older children.

18. Answer: C

The correct "incorrect" answer is pain is over-diagnosed and over-treated in hospitalized children. Pain is UNDER diagnosed and UNDER treated in children. Untreated pain will reinforce that painful procedures are punishment for misdeeds. The MOST important thing to do is to minimize separation from parents!

19. Answer: B

The correct answer is allow children to vent negative feelings. Parents should never take sides nor should they serve as referee! Parents should not use derogatory names and they should not permit verbal or physical abuse—neither is acceptable. Parents should encourage children to develop solutions and foster individuality in each child. They should spend time with each child individually. Also, it can be helpful to tell children about the conflicts that parents had themselves with their own siblings when they were children. Finally, define acceptable and unacceptable behavior.

20. Answer: D

The correct answer is encourage her mother to not use "don't" and "no" phrases. This child definitely needs to build her self-esteem! Ways to do this: Be an active listener and take interest in her activities. Use "positive" language—praise her for successes or achievements. It is best to discard labels, like "good" and "bad". Use encouragement as a tool to help her open up more. Overly protecting children will not help and will make things worse. So will focusing on mistakes. And you should suggest to the mother that she cannot expect perfection— this is undue pressure on the child and is likely aggravating the situation. While in the office, you would praise Jane for her good grades in school, or her pretty dress, or the way she smiles—provide appropriate behavior in front of the mother for her to model.

21. Answer: C

The correct answer is his fears should be validated, and to combat his fear of separation by a natural disaster, the parents should reassure him that they will all be together. This is one of those questions where you need to go for the "longest answer". I mean my goodness, would anyone write all that stuff out if it was a "wrong" answer?? Ok, back to the question. Remember these fears are quite common and require validation as well as reassurance to the child that the family will be together if it happens again—hopefully tornadoes won't, but earthquakes and bad lightening storms are going to recur depending on what part of the country the child lives. Children SHOULD be empowered to conquer their fears and physical examination is almost always normal. Laboratory studies are NOT indicated. It is important NOT to expose the child to more fear-provoking situations—like watching "The Wizard of Oz" or "Twister" is probably not a good idea!

22. Answer B

The correct answer is one month. Prevention in health care is at the core of pediatrics. Pediatricians spend as much as 40% of their day performing clinical preventive care from infancy through adolescence. Besides the traditional physical examination and immunizations, health supervision visits should include evaluation of developmental milestones, parent-infant interactions, anticipatory guidance, and a chance to answer questions for the family. The next visit for Mrs. Johnson's infant should occur at one month of age. The suggested post-natal schedule for health supervision visits is the first week of life followed by visits at one, two, four, six, nine, and twelve months of life.

23. Answer: A

The correct answer is MMR, IPV, and Varicella are all given as subcutaneous injections. DTaP, Hepatitis B, and *Haemophilus influenza* vaccines are given as intramuscular injections. I know this seems like a stupid question—but the ABP will expect you to know how these vaccines are given— many of the Peds residency programs require you personally to give the vaccines; so if you did, then you know this one cold—and certainly in a super busy clinical practice—most physicians don't do their own vaccines. Personally, I prefer to write the order and let the kid hate someone else <evil grin>.

24. Answer: C

The correct answer is she may administer the MMR vaccine but not the Varicella vaccine. After placing the Varicella vaccine into the syringe for administration it must be used within 30 minutes. The MMR can be given up to 8 hours after it is prepared. Note that waiting longer than 30 minutes is likely to diminish the potency of the vaccine. Some of us wonder if the reason why we see so many "breakthroughs" with the Varicella vaccine is the inappropriate handling in facilities providing the vaccine. It is one of the most labile vaccines that we give!

25. Answer: E

The correct answer is syncope. Syncope is actually quite common during/after vaccination, particularly in adolescents and younger adults. You should be on the look out for this particularly if pre syncopal manifestations occur—such as weakness or dizziness. In this particular case, the guy weighed 250lbs and was 6'3" tall. The nurse did not suffer any major damage.

26. Answer: A

The correct answer is the anterolateral aspect of the upper thigh and the deltoid region of the upper arm. Most of the manufacturers of vaccines will give flexibility in where the vaccine should be administered. However, these 2 sites are the most commonly used and recommended. The upper outer aspect of the buttocks is not a good site because the gluteal region is covered with a significant layer of subcutaneous fat and you may damage the sciatic nerve.

27. Answer: D

The correct answer is 1" for 4 month-old infant for thigh penetration; 2" for 130 kg male for deltoid penetration. Here the ABP wants you to realize that you have to use different size needles for different size children and locations of administration. The 2" cut off for adolescence applies to boys > 120 kg and girls >100 kg. 1" is going to be adequate for most children from 4-months to 70 kg. A 22 to 25-gauge needle is appropriate.

28. Answer: B

The correct answer is hepatitis B, DTaP, Hib, IPV. Hopefully this was an easy "gimme" question. The ABP sometimes can be nice and ask you these to give you a breather—they are rare so savor them for the moment—but don't take too much time—the next question is likely to be about some syndrome from Mars that you've never heard of.

29. Answer: D

The correct answer is if she has not had a history of varicella, she should receive 2 doses of vaccine, at least 1 month apart. Adolescents and young adults are at increased risk for complications from varicella and should be immunized appropriately if they are at risk. Children 13 and older require 2 doses spaced at least 1 month apart. Children younger than 13 only require 1 dose. Currently testing of adolescents and young adults is optional for positive serology—if she was positive then there would be no reason to give her vaccine. Positive titers = immunity. If she has a reliable history of varicella, then there also is no reason to vaccinate her.

30. Answer: A

The correct answer is DTaP, Hepatitis B, MMR, IPV. Since she is 5 years of age she does not require the Hib vaccine anymore. The pertussis component is currently not recommended for children older than 7 but this child is 5 so she still should receive it. All of the other vaccines are necessary and required. She would return in 1 month (4 weeks) to receive her next set of vaccines and also would receive varicella at that time if susceptible.

31. Answer: C

The correct answer is 4 weeks (1 month) for children "catching up" who are younger than 7 years of age. At that time she should receive DTaP, HBV, and Varicella (if susceptible). MMR could also be given, particularly if there were a community outbreak.

32. Answer: B

The correct answer is DTaP, HBV, Varicella. If there is a need (ie. outbreak in the community) she could receive her 2nd MMR then also. Since she is assumed susceptible to varicella she should receive that vaccine on her next visit.

33. Answer: A

The correct answer is hepatitis B, MMR, Td, IPV. Because he is older than 7 he does not require the pertussis component of the DTaP. Also, he doesn't require the larger "D" component of diphtheria at his age. Hib is not required for children older than 5 years of age. He does not require varicella vaccine. After he gets his immunizations today, when does he return? In 2 months—this is different than kids younger than 7 (one month for them!).

34. Answer: E

The correct answer is 8 weeks (2 months). Remember this is different for kids less than 7!!—they return in 1 month!

35. Answer: E

The correct answer is none, all of the vaccine pairs can be given at the same visit, without significantly diminishing immunogenicity.

36. Answer: A

The correct answer is none, she does not require reinstitution of the entire series for any of these vaccines. Since doses of all of these were missed at 4 and (for some) at 6 months, you would just start with her 2nd dose of each vaccine today. Then you would bring her back in the usual interval for the next dose of each vaccine.

37. Answer: B

The correct answer is reinstitute the entire immunization sequence for hepatitis B, polio, measles, mumps, rubella, diphtheria, and tetanus. In other words start over except for pertussis (she doesn't need if older than 7) and *Haemophilus influenzae* (doesn't need if older than 5). If she really is "up-to-date" then these "extra" vaccines will not be harmful to her. It is best to be sure that she is adequately protected!

38. Answer: D

The correct answer is to administer the MMR, IPV, and DTaP today. She is a well child otherwise and a minor upper respiratory infection is not a contraindication for vaccination. This is very clear in the ABP's mind!! Do not fail to give a vaccine to someone because of a minor illness. Remember that the minor illnesses and especially fever, do NOT interfere with the immunogenicity of the vaccine or increase the risk of side effects! Diarrheal illnesses are the same—they are not contraindications for vaccine. Other things that are not contraindications: current antimicrobial therapy, convalescent stage of illness, prematurity, pregnancy of the mother, recent exposure to an infectious disease, breast-feeding, allergies in relatives, allergies to penicillin, allergies to duck meat or feathers, family history of seizures, family history of sudden infant death syndrome, malnutrition. True contraindications are rare: anaphylaxis to neomycin or streptomycin—these are contained in some vaccines; previous anaphylaxis to a vaccine, severe reaction to a previous vaccine.

39. Answer: C

The correct answer is one recommendation is to feed both infants at the same time, with one on each breast. This would be ideal—however, babies may have different ideas as far as when they are hungry. The other recommendation, as in this case, would be to feed them at different times—of course if they are hungry at the same time then this wouldn't work either. Breast-feeding provides numerous benefits over bottle-feeding and in particular for the mother of twins, it is a HUGE economic benefit. If she is supplementing either or both twins with bottle feedings, then it is best NOT to prop the bottle, but for someone to hold the bottle. Most mothers of twins who attempt breast-feeding, with sufficient support and guidance, can do quite well. Interestingly, wet nurses have fed up to 6 infants at a time (ok..not ALL at the same time, but during a time period)—so supply of milk really isn't an issue. Timing and positioning of the infants is going to be the most important aspect for the new mother to work out.

40. Answer: E

The correct answer is all of the conditions listed are associated with high risks of maternal and perinatal morbidity/mortality.

41. Answer: D

The correct "incorrect" answer is in women who use steroidal contraceptives immediately before pregnancy; the date of conception is easily calculated. This is definitely FALSE. In these women, the EDC is likely to be completely unknown using menstrual history. All of the other methods listed are correct. Personally, I always liked to play with the little wheel thingee and figure out when I was conceived…OH that explains why the marriage date was on….Ok. Never mind.

42. Answer: A

The correct answer is urine culture. Asymptomatic bacteruria is quite common and should be treated with appropriate antibiotics. Without treatment, asymptomatic bacteruria can lead to acute pyelonephritis—actually it is pretty common in pregnant women—so you MUST do an initial urine culture during the initial prenatal visit. The acute pyelonephritis is then associated with increased risk of preterm labor and delivery. Other screening tests recommended: CBC (looking for anemia), Blood type and presence of any maternal antibody to red blood cell antigens, VDRL or RPR for syphilis, Rubella titers to confirm immunity, a urinalysis to screen for glucose and protein, and HIV testing should be offered—since we have effective means to prevent transmission to the infant.

43. Answer: B

The correct answer is prepregnancy height of <150 cm (essentially less than 5 ft tall). There is increased risk of preterm labor for women who are younger than 18 as well as if they have a prepregnancy weight LESS than 45 kg (less than 100 lbs). Previous abdominal surgery does not generally put a woman at increased risk—but abdominal surgery *during* the pregnancy would. Previous oral contraceptive use does not cause any increased risk either. Other factors: low socioeconomic status, "work outside the home"—this was published in texts in the 90s; still—it makes you wonder if it is still true today?, cigarette smoking (>10 cigarettes a day).

44. Answer: C

The correct answer is bilateral cryptorchidism. Prune-belly syndrome occurs in 1 in 40,000 live births, 95% of affected individuals are male. It is commonly associated with deficient abdominal muscles, bilateral undescended testicles, and urinary tract anomalies. Oligohydramnios and pulmonary hypoplasia may be associated. Malrotation of the bowel, musculoskeletal abnormalities, and cardiac abnormalities may be associated. Low set ears, micrognathia, and microcephaly have not been associated with this disorder. Orchiopexy should be attempted in the first six months of life.

45. Answer: B

The correct answer is active, untreated tuberculosis. All of the other items listed are safe for the mother to breast feed—even acute rubella infection! She is more likely to transmit Rubella via other means than breast-feeding.

46. Answer: D

The correct answer is metronidazole. It is contraindicated for the mother who is breast-feeding. If she must take the drug, then it is recommended that she stop breast-feeding while on the medication. She can resume breast-feeding 24 hours after her last dose. The other agents are compatible with breast-feeding. Isoniazid appears to be safe and although hepatotoxicity is a concern, it has not been documented. Usually, the infant will also be placed on pyridoxine while the mother is on therapy.

47. Answer: C

The correct answer is the first 28 days of life. This is the "neonatal" period. This is the SINGLE most important period of childhood during which the HIGHEST mortality occurs. Also "lifetime" morbidity from "neonatal" occurring events is also frequent.

48. Answer: A

The correct answer is a Caucasian Male. This group of the general population in the United States has the highest mortality rate across the birthweight spectrum for infants.

49. Answer: B

The correct answer is vigorous cry. Most newborns at birth will cry vigorously and tend to remain awake for about a half hour or so. A feeble or soft cry is abnormal as is a high-pitched or shrieking cry—these suggest a neurological problem. A hoarse cry suggests vocal cord paralysis, hypothyroidism, or trauma to the hypopharynx.

50. Answer: E

The correct answer is smooth soles without creases. Creases in the soles do not appear until about 32-33 weeks. All the other findings are consistent with a child older than 32 weeks.

51. Answer: C

The correct answer is dry, peeling skin and less than normal subcutaneous tissue. In the post-term infant, he/she will appear alert but have a "wasted" appearance with dry, peeling skin and less than normal subcutaneous tissues. The fingernails will be very long (well past the finger tips) and there may be meconium staining of the skin, cord, and nails.

52. Answer: E

The correct answer is there is no pathological significance associated with this finding. This is known as *Harlequinism*. It is a transient change in the color of the skin of the newborn in which one side of the body turns red and the other side remains pale. It is sharply demarcated at the midline. The changes can last for only a few seconds to several minutes. It can recur but has no pathological significance.

53. Answer: B

The correct answer is an immediate work-up should ensue particularly for hemolytic anemia. Jaundice appearing in the first 24 hours is rarely normal. Usually it is due to a hemolytic process or breakdown of a large hematoma.

54. Answer: A

The correct answer is drug withdrawal. This is associated with tachycardia. Other things associated with tachycardia in the newborn period include fever, hypovolemia, congenital heart disease, tachyarrhythmias, anemia, and hyperthyroidism. All of the other items in the question are associated with bradycardia. Bradycardia in newborns is generally defined as a persistent heart rate of 80 beats (or less) per minute.

55. Answer: D

The correct answer is penile length of 2 cm. Any penile length less than 2.5 cm requires endocrinologic evaluation. The spleen tip is usually palpable to just below the left costal margin—if it is more than 1 cm, that is considered abnormal. The liver can be palpable up to 3 cm in the normal infant. The labia majora usually do meet in the midline and can obscure both the urethra and clitoris. The lower portion of each kidney is palpable—particularly during the 1st day of life before the bowel is filled with gas.

56. Answer: D

The correct answer is the cord can be covered with a moist dressing to promote healing. The cord should be allowed to air dry and be swabbed daily with alcohol. Covering the cord with a moist or occlusive dressing will serve to set up the area as "a culture media" for microorganisms. Antiseptics and antibiotics are also usually not necessary in routine cord care. All of the other choices listed are appropriate for routine newborn care.

57. Answer: D

The answer is this is a normal phase, and she should continue offering a variety of foods without forcing the child to eat. Most children will have a decrease in appetite around the end of the first year and during the second year due to decreased rate of growth. Their caloric intake per kg of body weight therefore decreases. If offered a variety of foods, children will, over several days, select foods that make up a balanced diet. Forcing a child at this age to eat causes stress, and the child usually rebels--causing feeding problems. Increasing snacks or the amount of milk will only cause the child to feel even less hungry and less likely to eat meals.

58. Answer: C

The correct answer is phenylalanine by tyrosine. The 9 essential amino acids are: Leucine, Isoleucine, Lysine, Methionine, Phenylalanine, Threonine, Tryptophan, Valine, and Histidine. Ok---this one you should have been able to figure out without any knowledge of this junk (I mean important clinical information of course!). What do diet drinks have in them? Phenylalanine! And we know that people with PKU deficiency cannot take this, right? Therefore, somehow humans are able to utilize another amino acid instead. And PKU deficient patients who cannot tolerate phenylalanine in their diets (and therefore don't have any phenylalanine available) can substitute tyrosine instead. The other substitution occurs when methionine can be substituted by cysteine.

59. Answer: A

The correct answer is the newborn infant. They require 1.5 to 2 grams/kg/day and this gradually decreases over time. A 6-12 month old infant requires 1.5 grams/kg/day. During early childhood this reduces to 1 g/kg/day. Older children require even less. Adolescents experiencing a growth spurt can see this return to 1 gram/kg/day. Finally, adults only require 0.8 gm/kg/day.

60. Answer: B

The correct answer is 9 kcal/g. Now just memorize this. Fats have 9 kcal/kg of potential energy while carbohydrates and protein essentially have about 4 kcal/kg. This always seems to appear on Board exams—not sure why..but it does!! Dietary fat is the highest density source of potential energy. Fats are often considered bad—but they provide important nutritional functions: store energy as adipose tissue (wow--glad this is good—I've got a lot of stored energy!); provide essential micronutrients—essential fatty acids like linoleic acid; facilitate absorption and transportation of fat soluble vitamins; and enhance the appeal of food—by their aroma and taste.

61. Answer: E

The correct answer is all of the choices are true. Remember that we have endogenous de novo biosynthesis (mainly in the liver) as well as exogenous sources. Unfortunately dietary changes in cholesterol intake really only make minor changes in total plasma cholesterol—thus the burgeoning expansion of the anti-lipid agents available for adults today.

62. Answer: A

The correct "incorrect" answer is high levels of linoleic acid. Essential fatty acid deficiency is defined biochemically as low levels of linoleic acid sufficient to alter fatty acid metabolism. Remember, linoleic acid is THE main essential fatty acid. Classically there is a decrease in arachidonic acid levels and the clinical manifestations may present as listed in the choices. Certain groups of children may develop fatty acid deficiency including those with cystic fibrosis and infants with hepatobiliary disease. Also, any child or infant that is on parenteral hyperalimentation that does not include lipid is at risk for developing linoleic acid deficiency.

63. Answer: C

The correct answer is TBW decreases, ICW increases, and ECW decreases. At birth TBW is 80%, ICW is 35% and ECW is 45%. By 10 years of age, TBW has decreased to 60%, ICW has increased to 40%, and ECW decreases to 20%.

64. Answer: E

The correct answer is 1000 ml of 5% dextrose IV to which 40mEq of potassium chloride and 57 mEq of sodium is added. Let's calculate this out. We assume that normal maintenance therapy for a child with a caloric expenditure of 500 kcal is needed. The infant's total body fluid deficit is calculated by 5kg x 10% = 500 mL. This represents ECF, which is 60% of the 500ml, and ICF, which is 40% of the 500 ml. So the ECF deficit is 500 ml x 60% = 300 ml. The ICF deficit is 500 ml x 40% = 200 mL. So for the amount of fluid we need: 500 (maintenance) + 500 ml deficit = 1000 ml.

Now what about those sodium and potassium values? How did we get those?

Well for the ECF: we have 300 ml deficit. Thus 300 mL/1000ml x 140 mEq/L gives us a value of 42 mEq of sodium and 300ml/1000ml x 100 mEq/L of chloride = 30mEq of chloride. In the ICF the 200mL should contain 200 ml/1000mL x 150 mEq/L = 30 mEq of potassium.

For maintenance fluid remember that for every 1L you have 30 mEq of Sodium, 20 mEq of potassium and 20 mEq of Chloride. So with a 500 ml maintenance we would need 15 mEq of Sodium, 10 mEq of potassium and 10 mEq of chloride.

So we add the Maintenance electrolytes to the deficit electrolytes and get for Sodium: 15 mEq + 42 mEq = 57 mEq. And for the Potassium: 10 mEq + 30 mEq = 40 mEq of potassium.

So, the child needs 1000ml of 5% dextrose IV to which 40 mEq of potassium chloride and 57 mEq of sodium with appropriate anions (usually is chloride) have been added.

65. Answer: B

The correct answer is 2850 mL. First, what is his maintenance requirement?

He is 25 kg:

First 10 kg = 1000 ml
Next 10 kg= 500 ml
20 ml x 5 kg = 100 ml

Total Maintenance: 1600 mL

Now his deficit:
5% x 25 kg = .05 x 25,000 mL = 1250 mL

So his total requirement for the next 24 hours would be 1250 mL + 1600 mL = 2850 mL.

66. Answer: D

The correct answer is 81 mEq. Ok—she has hypotonic dehydration (the serum Na of 120 mEq/L tells us this!).

First, how much does she need for maintenance? Remember 30mEq/L is maintenance for this age. So, what is her maintenance fluid requirement? 5 kg x 100 ml = 500 ml. So she will need 15 mEq of sodium for maintenance.

Now what is her deficit? We want to get her sodium to 135 mEq. So she is 15 mEq below that now (135-120). We know that .6mEq of sodium per kg body weight will increase the serum sodium concentration by 1 mEq/L—so we use the formula:

NaCl required = (135 − observed serum Na) x 0.6 x weight (kg)

NaCl required = (135 − 120) x 0.6 x 5 = 15 x 0.6 x 5 = 45 mEq of NaCl additional required.

So, Maintenance + additional = 15 mEq + 45 mEq = 60 mEq NaCl. BUT WAIT!! We forgot about the ECF deficit that is not included in the sodium we have calculated.

Remember that maintenance water is 500 ml. And her deficit water calculation is 5 kg x 5% = 5000 ml x .05 = 250 mL.

Of this 250 ml how much is ECF (which, remember, this is the part of the body that contains Na)? So we calculate: 250 mL x .6 = 150 ml

So how much Sodium is required in 150 ml of ECF for replacement? 150ml/1000mL x 140 mEq/L = 21 mEq of Sodium.

So, now we add 21 mEq to our Maintenance (15 mEq) and to our extra replacement (45 mEq): 21 + 15 + 45 = 81 mEq of Sodium.

67. Answer: A

The correct answer is 1000 ml total, 175 ml "free" water. Let's figure out the Total water requirement first:

Normal maintenance for her is 100 ml x 5 kg = 500 ml.

Now her deficit is 10% or 5000 ml x .1 = 500 ml

So her total fluid required will be 1000 ml (500 + 500).

Of the 500 ml that is deficit, how much should be "free" water (ie. without electrolytes)? The recommendations are to give 1/3 of the deficit as "free" water in severe hypertonic dehydration. So, 1/3 of 500 ml is approximately 175 ml. So, of the total 1000 ml, 175 ml would be 5% dextrose without electrolytes added to the bag. The remaining 325 ml is calculated based on the usual deficit numbers—60% will be ECF replacement (200 ml) and 40% will be ICF replacement (125 ml). The 325 ml will contain electrolytes corresponding to the individual compartments we are replacing.

68. Answer: D

The correct answer is fluoride supplementation. Fluoride does not pass into human milk in significant amounts regardless of the mother's fluoride intake. Therefore, a fluoride supplement is recommended for the breast-fed infant shortly after birth, or no later than 6 months of age. Vitamin D could be required if the child was not given fluoride supplementation and was NOT exposed to sunlight.

69. Answer: C

The correct answer is 6 months of age. Iron stores become depleted after 4-6 months of age. Human milk and non-fortified infant formula do not contain enough iron for nutritional purposes. Most children are given an iron-fortified cereal, which usually provides about 1.6 mg of iron per tablespoon. They can also be placed on iron drops.

70. Answer: B

The correct answer is Stimulate absorption of calcium and phosphorus from the small intestine and reabsorption of calcium from the kidney. Vitamin D undergoes hydroxylation to 25-hyrdoxyvitamin D in the liver and 1-α-hydroxylation in the kidney to 1, 25-dihyroxyvitamin D (1, 25 $(OH)_2D$--a true hormone).

71. Answer: E

The correct answer is necrotizing enterocolitis (NEC). This should have been pretty obvious. The gut is in a state of complete shutdown—there is no way you would want to give enteral feeds in this state. The cells of the lining of the small and large intestines are barely able to function to sustain themselves—let alone carry out complex absorption and secretion processes. Gut rest is mandatory for NEC. Other conditions that are contraindicated: adynamic ileus, persistent vomiting, severe respiratory distress, upper GI bleeding, and intestinal obstruction.

72. Answer: C

The correct answer is lower incisor position. These can be either supernumerary teeth or true, deciduous "milk" teeth. If they are loose or if they are painful for the mother during breastfeeding they can be removed—however, if they are true deciduous teeth they will leave a gap for at least 7 years until the permanent teeth appear. This could be a problem for positioning of the molars and dental arch.

73. Answer: B

The correct answer is mandibular central incisors, maxillary central incisors, and then second molars. The mandibular teeth generally erupt before the maxillary teeth. The same holds true for permanent teeth eruption.

74. Answer: C

The correct answer is 6 to 8. Kids this age don't have permanent teeth erupting yet. Generally, permanent tooth eruption occurs at age 6-7 years.

75. Answer: E

The correct answer is dentinogenesis imperfecta (hereditary opalescent dentin). The findings described in the question are "classic" for this condition. It occurs in 1/8000 people and is the most frequent inheritable disorder of dental structure. It can occur with osteogenesis imperfecta. Ellis-van Creveld syndrome is a weird syndrome with severe respiratory distress resulting from pulmonary hypoplasia and a narrow dysplastic thorax with extremely short ribs. They may have natal teeth as well as too few or too many teeth. Cherubism is a familial fibro-osseous disease that involves the jaws. The initial appearance is unilateral fullness of the cheek in the 2nd or 3rd years of life. The disease regresses over time and the lesions dissipate. Hallermann-Streiff syndrome is an obscure disease that is just in a table in one of the standard Peds Texts. It is associated with a small, hypoplastic mandible, microphthalmia, cataracts and neonatal teeth.

76. Answer: C

The correct answer is the first molars. They usually erupt between the ages of 6 and 7 years. These molars are very important for future structural development of the mouth. They maintain the dental arch in place when the primary molars are lost.

77. Answer: B

The answer is Glycogen Storage Disease type IIA (Pompe disease). Pompe disease is inherited as an autosomal recessive disorder causing deficient activity of alpha-glucosidase. This results in accumulation of glycogen in muscle, liver, heart, kidney, smooth muscle, and nerves. This is just about the only condition in which there is such marked hypotonia and cardiomegaly in an infant who was normal at birth.

These infants present with muscle weakness, hepatomegaly, severe cardiomegaly, and normal mental development. They have normal blood glucose unlike von Gierke disease. The EKG findings of shortened PR intervals and massive QRS complexes are typical for the disease.

There is no specific treatment, and death usually occurs within 2 years of age.

78. Answer: D

The answer is William's syndrome. These children have short stature, mental retardation, friendly loquacious personality, and hoarse voice. The facies of the patient described is typical as well as epicanthal folds, blue eyes with stellate pattern in iris. The murmur described is that of supravalvular aortic stenosis which is commonly found in William's syndrome, although other heart defects may also be seen. The syndrome is caused by deletion of one elastin allele located on chromosome 7q11.23.

79. Answer: B

The answer is evaluation of the adrenal axis. The described infant likely has Down's syndrome (DS) as manifested by a protruding tongue, hypotonia, evidence of duodenal atresia and birth to a mother of advanced age. Several major anomalies are associated with DS including cardiac defects (45%) (AV canal defects, VSD, hypoplastic left heart) and duodenal atresia (7%). Hypothyroidism and neonatal/infant leukemia (15X more frequent) are also seen at increased frequency in this population of children. Mental retardation is universal with only rare exceptions, although with appropriate early childhood experiences, > 95% can attain a level of semi-independent living by adulthood. No increase in adrenal disease has been described in DS children compared with normal counterparts.

80. Answer: D

The answer is perinatal exposure to methotrexate. The features described are consistent with Trisomy 13 or 18 Syndrome, which are rare chromosomal disorders with frequent phenotypic overlap. Most chromosomal errors are a result of meiotic nondisjunction, and the risk increases with advancing maternal age, as in Down's syndrome. However, 20% of live-born infants have the characteristic phenotype but normal chromosomes, which may result from a single gene dominant mutation or autosomal recessive inheritance. In the case described, however, prenatal diagnosis of maternal Crohn Disease raises the likelihood the mother was treated with methotrexate during pregnancy, an agent well-known for causing the abnormal phenotype seen in Trisomy 13/18.

21q22.2-22.3 cryptic chromosomal rearrangements are seen in cases of Down's syndrome with normal chromosome number. Excess CGG repeats on the X chromosome result in the Fragile X Syndrome. The Trisomy 13/18 phenotype is not associated with prenatal exposure to sulfasalazine.

81. Answer: A

The answer is full chromosomal analysis and echocardiography. This patient likely has a mosaic presentation of Turner's Syndrome (TS). 15% of individuals with TS are mosaics with chromosomes reflecting XO/XX, XO/XX/XXX or XO/XY genotypes. In this subset, many have muted features and often are fertile. Sometimes the diagnosis escapes physicians when the patients are phenotypically normal except for short stature. The majority of patients with TS (60%) will have the 45 XO genotype and demonstrate primary amenorrhea, sterility, sparse pubic/axillary hair, underdeveloped breasts and short stature. The remaining 25% of patients will have a 46XX genotype but one X chromosome will be structurally abnormal (short arm deletion, for example). These patients have a higher incidence of associated serious major anomalies, including mental retardation.

In general, all patients with TS are at increased risk for coarctation of the aorta (15%) and any patient with a phenotype suspicious for TS should be referred for echocardiography if the blood pressure is elevated. 75% of patients with TS demonstrate normal intelligence and can achieve some secondary sexual characteristics if treated with adequate hormonal therapy during adolescence.

The diagnosis is made by full chromosomal analysis, as buccal smears may be positive for sex chromatin in mosaics and patients with a structurally abnormal X chromosome resulting in a falsely negative test for TS.

---

82. Answer: D

The answer is the infant has clinical features suggestive of Smith-Lemli-Opitz Syndrome and may have concomitant hypospadias, congenital heart disease and death by 18 months of age. SLOS is an autosomal recessive disorder presenting as 1 in 20,000 live births. Defective cholesterol biosynthesis with cholesterol deficiency and accumulation of potentially toxic cholesterol precursor molecules is hypothesized as the etiology of defective CNS myelination and cataract formation. Patients present as SGA infants with microcephaly, a prominent occiput and narrow frontal area, eyelid ptosis, epicanthal folds, strabismus, low-set or posteriorly rotated ears, broad nasal tip with upturned nares, micrognathia, simian creases, syndactyly of 2nd and 3rd toes, hypospadias with cryptorchidism or ambiguous genitalia, clenched hand abnormalities, cleft palate, bifid uvula, structural abnormalities of the CNS with or without seizures, hypoplastic left heart and multiple gastrointestinal and renal anomalies. Hypotonia eventually may progress to hypertonia with irritability, shrill screaming, feeding problems and failure to thrive. Prognosis is poor, even with cholesterol therapy, with 80% of infants dying by age 18 months. Risk for recurrence in a couple with an affected child is 25% due to the classical Mendelian autosomal recessive inheritance pattern.

Many of the features of SLOS are shared with Trisomy 18, but patients with Trisomy 18 do not have normal intelligence. Some infants with phenotypes of Trisomy 18 have normal chromosomes and are considered variants of SLOS.

While infants with Down's Syndrome may also have simian creases, epicanthal folds and congenital heart disease (hypoplastic left heart, AV canal defects, VSDs), the phenotype of Down's Syndrome patients is somewhat different and includes upward slanting eyes, Brushfield spots, a small upturned nose with a saddle bridge, a small mouth with protruding tongue, a short neck with redundant skin folds, clinodactyly of 5th fingers and a wide space between the 1st and 2nd toes. Hypotonia during infancy is notable in DS, but does not progress to hypertonia with associated irritability as in SLOS. With directive medical care, DS patients live into adulthood.

Noonan's Syndrome is characterized by many of the features of Turner's syndrome: short stature, web neck, low posterior hairline, broad chest with wide-spaced nipples, peripheral edema and cardiac defects. Pulmonary stenosis is the most commonly observed cardiac defect associated with Noonan's syndrome. The disorder is marked by mental deficiency with normal chromosomes.

Trisomy 2 is not compatible with life.

83. Answer: C

The correct answer is to order serum organic acids. Neonates with metabolic abnormalities are often normal at birth. They subsequently may present with signs and symptoms that are clinically indistinguishable from sepsis including metabolic acidosis, vomiting, lethargy, and poor feeding. Metabolic derangements that present with clinical manifestations at such an early age are very often lethal if not quickly diagnosed and specifically treated. In this child, sepsis must be considered. However, the index of suspicion for an inborn error of metabolism should be high in this patient. The odor in the room, the lack of fever, and the normal blood pressure are clues that diagnoses other than sepsis should be considered. When a metabolic disturbance is suspected in the presence of a metabolic acidosis with normal ammonia levels, an organic acidemia should be suspected. Serum organic acids should be measured in addition to a complete septic evaluation. Serum aminoacidopathies do not typically cause a metabolic acidosis.

84. Answer: A

The correct answer is urea cycle defect. Neonates with metabolic abnormalities are often normal at birth. They subsequently may present with signs and symptoms that may include metabolic acidosis, vomiting, lethargy, and poor feeding.   Vomiting may be severe and projectile, sometimes arousing suspicion for pyloric stenosis. Metabolic derangements that present with clinical manifestations at such an early age are very often lethal if not quickly diagnosed and specifically treated. The most common cause of hyperammonemia in infants is a defect in the urea cycle. Infants with urea cycle defects typically have normal serum pH and bicarbonate levels. Organic acidemia typically causes a metabolic acidosis. Serum amino acidemias typically produce normal ammonia levels.

85. Answer: C

The correct answer is intermittent maple syrup urine disease. Neonates with metabolic abnormalities are often normal at birth. They subsequently may present with signs and symptoms that are clinically indistinguishable from sepsis including metabolic acidosis, vomiting, lethargy, and poor feeding. Metabolic derangements that present with clinical manifestations at such an early age are very often lethal if not quickly diagnosed and specifically treated. In this child, sepsis must be considered. However, the index of suspicion for an inborn error of metabolism should be high in this patient. The odor in the room, the lack of fever, and the normal blood pressure are clues that diagnoses other than sepsis should be considered. In intermittent maple syrup urine disease, previously normal infants and children develop the classic symptoms of MSUD during times of stress, including illnesses and surgery. These symptoms include vomiting, an aroma of maple syrup, and lethargy. This may progress to coma and death. Urea cycle defects typically produce elevated ammonia levels with normal serum pH and bicarbonate levels.

86. Answer: B

The correct answer is intravenous administration of a glucose containing solution. The baby has Glycogen storage disease 1b. Patients with this disorder typically present in the third or fourth month of life with signs and symptoms of hypoglycemia, lactic acidosis, and hepatomegaly. Associated inflammatory bowel disease as well as associated abnormalities of platelet adhesion may contribute to GI blood loss. The astute clinician will recognize that hypoglycemia is the likely etiology of this child's seizure. Intramuscular administration of glucagon will result in increased lactate levels and not glycogenolysis in this patient. Hyponatremia and hypocalcemia are not features of this disorder. Thus, administration of 3%NaCl or Calcium Gluconate are not indicated and may be harmful. An anticonvulsant medication such as fosphenytoin sodium may lack efficacy as long as the underlying etiology is not corrected.

87. Answer: E

The correct answer is serum glycine level. This child has neonatal non-ketotic hyperglycinemia (NKH). This disorder presents with perinatal intractable myoclonic seizures, hiccups, lethargy, hypotonia, apnea, and poor feeding. Elevated glycine level may be found in the blood, urine, and CSF. There is no acidemia. Treatment is supportive. Surviving infants typically experience profound psychomotor retardation and an intractable seizure disorder. Serum lactate levels and serum ketone levels should not be elevated in the absence of metabolic acidosis. Viral cultures are not indicated.

88. Answer: C

The correct answer is administration of carnitine. This patient has medium chain Acyl CoA dehydrogenase deficiency (MCAD). MCAD typically presents with a hypoketotic hypoglycemia and a Reyes-like illness during the first three years of life. Vomiting, lethargy, coma, and circulatory collapse may occur. There is little or no acidemia unless it is related to the triggering disorder, as in diarrhea in this patient. Plasma and tissue carnitine levels are low. Acute illness is triggered by a fasting state for more than 12 hours as may occur with an acute gastroenteritis. Although sepsis must be considered in this patient, broader antibiotic coverage is not indicated. There is no indication for the administration of biotin or thiamine. Exchange transfusion is not helpful in the treatment of MCAD.

89. Answer: B

The correct answer is debranching enzyme deficiency (Type III). These patients have a generally good prognosis. Most will improve by adolescence and will be asymptomatic by then. Patients with von Gierke's disease and glucose-6-phoshatase microsomal transport defect usually die before the age of 2 from ketoacidosis or other complications. Those with Pompe's die in early infancy due to cardiac failure because of the cardiac muscle involvement. Those with brancher enzyme deficiency frequently die before their 10th birthday due to hepatic cirrhosis.

90. Answer: E

The correct answer is 13q-. 20-30% of those affected will have retinoblastoma. Other features with this autosomal syndrome: prenatal growth deficiency, high nasal bridge and protruding maxilla, thumb hypoplasia or absence and congenital heart disease (nearly 50%). Imperforate anus is also associated with this.

91. Answer: A

The correct answer is "cat cry". This is the classic "cri du chat" syndrome. These children have severe mental retardation with round face, down-slanted palpebral fissures and a simian crease. 30% will have congenital heart disease. The "cat cry" occurs in infancy and they develop premature graying in adolescence.

92. Answer: D

The correct answer is webbed neck. Children with 4p- deficiency have all of the other findings listed. Seizures occur in 50% and a scalp defect occurs in 10% or so. Hypospadias occurs in males and cleft lip is seen in 50%. Webbed neck is seen in 18p- and Turner's syndrome.

93. Answer: C

The correct answer is isolated extra digit. Generally one primary malformation without significance can be "observed" before doing a significant workup. The other items listed generally would warrant a cytogenetic analysis. On the boards, look out for infants with multiple dysmorphic features—these you want to work up! Also if they give you "keyword" clues—like "webbed neck" or a girl with short stature and amenorrhea!

94. Answer: D

The correct answer is over 80% are due to 47 XX7, 47 XYY and 47 XXX. The phenotypic alterations in XO are usually apparent—webbed neck, short stature and amenorrhea. 1/500 of live-born infants have an abnormality of the sex chromosomes. 47 XXY are phenotypically male (this is Klinefelter's syndrome). 47 XYY are men who have tall stature characteristically.

95. Answer: C

The correct answer is phenylalanine cannot be converted to tyrosine and phenylpyruvic acid is excreted in the urine. The classic characteristic in untreated patients is severe mental retardation (IQ < 30). PKU infants appear normal at birth, but early symptoms occur in about ½. They develop a characteristic "mousy", barn-like odor. Physical development is normal and they usually are cute children. It occurs in 1/10,000 to 1/20,000. It is autosomal recessive. Treatment is with a diet low in phenylalanine. Even infants with PKU require a certain amount of phenylalanine in their diet!

96. Answer: A

The correct answer is alkaptonuria. This results from a defect in the enzyme homogentisic acid oxidase and is characterized by the excretion of dark-colored urine. It is an autosomal recessive disorder. Frequently the urine is "normal" in color and on standing or alkalinization is turns dark brown or black. The urine gives a positive test for reducing substance and a positive ferric chloride test. Alkaptonuria can be demonstrated by exposing undeveloped photographic film to urine—which immediately blackens it—wow, what a great party trick! People with this disease are usually asymptomatic in childhood. Adults in their 40s will deposit brownish or bluish pigment on their ears or sclerae. The deposition of pigment maybe extensive and is known as ochronosis. Arthritis can occur later and can resemble rheumatoid or osteoarthritis.

97. Answer: E

The correct answer is he is unable to metabolize leucine, isoleucine, and valine properly. These are the "branched-chain" amino acids. He has Maple Syrup Urine disease. This leads to high concentrations of these amino acids in the blood and urine as well as the ketoacid analogs in the urine. This is an autosomal recessive disorder. Most patients by the time they present have permanent brain damage.

98. Answer: D

The answer is: metachromatic leukodystrophy (MLD). It is caused by a deficiency of arylsulfatase A (ASA) and is inherited as an autosomal recessive disorder. ASA is needed for the hydrolysis of sulfated glycosphingolipids, and when deficient, results in white matter storage of these glycosphingolipids. This leads to demyelination and a neurodegenerative course.

The most common form usually presents between age 12-18 months with difficulty walking and genu recurvatum. Deep tendon reflexes are diminished or absent. Myoclonic seizures, dementia and spastic paraplegia are followed by death in the first decade of life.

The juvenile (presenting as late as 20 years of age) and the adult (presenting after the second decade) forms present with ataxia, spasticity, and decreased deep tendon reflexes followed by seizures, dementia and spastic quadriplegia. The psychiatric manifestations are more prominent in the adult form.

MLD should be suspected in patients with the above-mentioned symptoms. Metachromatic deposits in biopsied segments of the sural nerve, metachromatic granules in urinary sediment, decreased nerve conduction velocities, and increased spinal fluid protein all suggest MLD. The diagnosis is confirmed by demonstrating decreased activity of arylsulfatase A in leukocytes of skin fibroblasts. Supportive therapy is the primary intervention.

99. Answer: E

The answer is: Fabry disease. It is caused by deficiency of α-galactosidase A resulting in storage of glycosphingolipids in the plasma and lysosomes of vascular endothelial and smooth muscle cells. It is inherited as X-linked recessive and characterized by angiokeratomas (most dense in the "bathing trunk area"), hypohidrosis, corneal opacities, acroparesthesias, and vascular disease of the heart, kidneys, and/or brain. With increasing age, the vascular disease leads to major morbidity including heart and renal dysfunction.

The diagnosis is usually made from the history and the characteristic skin lesions and eye findings. It is confirmed by demonstrating decreased α-galactosidase A activity in plasma, leukocytes, or cultured fibroblasts.

Treatment consists of phenytoin and carbamazepine for pain control and supportive care. Dialysis or renal transplant is used for renal dysfunction.

100. Answer: A

The correct answer is measure galactose-1-phosphate uridyl transferase in red blood cells. This is the best way to confirm the diagnosis. Galactosuria does not confirm the diagnosis as this can also occur in galactokinase deficiency also.

101. Answer: C

The correct answer is she will become symptomatic if she is fed cow's milk or breast milk. She cannot tolerate lactose-containing agents—lactose is broken down into glucose and galactose—which she cannot metabolize. She must be fed a galactose free-diet. Since lactose is really the only naturally occurring form of galactose, it is not that difficult.

102. Answer: C

The correct answer is 303 mOsm/L. Use (2 x Na) + BUN/2.8 + Glucose/18. A "quick and dirty" estimate is (2 x Na) + BUN/3 Glucose/20. The more "precise" method gives you (2 x 120) + 21/2.8 + 1000/18 = 303 mOsm/L. The "estimated" quick and dirty gives you (2 x 120) + 21/3 + 1000/20 = 297 mOsm/L. 297 is closest to 303—nothing else is even close-286 was 11 mOsm/L away.

103. Answer: D

The correct answer is mandatory in all states by law. It occurs in 1/10,000 births.

104. Answer: D

The correct answer is massive cardiomegaly, congestive heart failure, and early death (usually in infancy). ECG usually shows very large QRS complexes and a shortened P-R interval.

105. Answer: A

The correct answer is look for an inborn error of leucine catabolism caused by a deficiency of isovaleryl-coenzyme A dehydrogenase. Isovaleric acid is the principal metabolite causing the "sweaty feet" odor in isovaleric acidemia. The key here—go for the long answer!! I wouldn't waste my time writing out this junk (I mean, important information) otherwise. Actually this is one of their favorites..so..put "sweaty feet" with leucine catabolism and you will be on the right track. Another way I remember it is: think of Lucy (leucine) and Valerie (isovaleric) having a fight..and they get all sweaty..Ok, it may not be much help to you—but it brings up some interesting images…

106. Answer: D

The correct answer is methylcrotonylgycinuria (methylcrotonyl-CoA carboxylase deficiency). Not much exciting with this deficiency except this little tidbit. Personally I haven't smelled much cat urine in my life—but then again I've still got something to look forward to I guess in my old age.

107. Answer: C

The correct answer is D-penicillamine. D-penicillamine has sulfhydryl-containing amino acid and forms disulfides which are excreted with free cysteine, thereby decreasing the concentration of cystine in the urine. Increased water intake is recommended, NOT restriction, to help with diuresis of the cystine.

108. Answer: B

The correct answer is classic compulsive self-destructive behavior occurs after 18 months of age. This is an X-linked recessive disorder so this is a male-only disorder. Infants usually are asymptomatic at birth but by 3-4 months of age show signs of vomiting, hypotonia and delayed motor development. Dystonia, chorea, and athetosis appear usually between 6 months and 1 year. Between 1 and 2 years of age the children show increasing spasticity, dysarthria and inability to ambulate. By 18 months of age, they show classic compulsive self-destructive behavior including lip mutilation, finger-biting, and head-banging. The urine uric acid/creatinine ratio is markedly elevated in affected children.

109. Answer: D

The correct answer is hypophosphatemia. It can occur within a few minutes of eating fructose and occurs before clinical symptoms appear. Hypoglycemia and severe gastrointestinal distress occur soon after the hypophosphatemia develops.

110. Answer: A

The correct answer is Type IIa. Type I, IV, and V can cause xanthomas but type IIa most commonly causes xanthomas of tendons. Type IIb does not cause xanthomas at all.

111. Answer: C

The correct answer is Wilson's disease. The picture shows you classic Kayser-Fleischer rings, the yellowish-brown discoloration in the cornea close to the limbus. It can present many ways but a chronic hepatitis-like picture is common. Multiple organs can be involved due to the excess amount of copper. This is an autosomal recessive disorder of copper metabolism. A mutated copper-transporting enzyme prevents the excretion of copper detached from the copper-transporting ceruloplasmin into the bile. Rising copper levels inhibit ceruloplasmin formation from apo-ceruloplasmin. A marker for this disease is a low ceruloplasmin but remember that the low ceruloplasmin does NOT cause the disease process, it is the excess copper. By the way, the Cross-Hannaman syndrome does not exist but if it did it would mean you were really cool.

112. Answer: A

The correct answer is abetalipoproteinemia. This disorder is classified as absence of the beta lipoproteins in plasma. These patients have failure to thrive and have a "spiny" appearance to their red blood cells on peripheral smear (acanthocytosis). They also have ataxia and develop retinitis pigmentosa.

113. Answer: B

The correct "incorrect" answer is nervous system involvement is common. Actually the nervous system is usually NOT involved. All of the other items listed are true.

114. Answer: D

The correct answer is Hurler's syndrome (type I mucopolysaccharidosis). All of the features described go along with this syndrome. Other features include hydrocephalus, myocardial dysfunction, and infiltration of the mitral and aortic valves with mucopolysaccharide. The disease is due to a deficiency in alpha-L-iduronidase which is required for the degradation of both dermatan sulfate and heparin sulfate. These substances would be found in the urine and would help make the diagnosis if found.

115. Answer: E

The correct answer is dermatan and heparin sulfate. The disease is due to a deficiency in alpha-L-iduronidase which is required for the degradation of both dermatan sulfate and heparin sulfate. These substances would be found in the urine and would help make the diagnosis if found.

116. Answer: C

The correct answer is cirrhosis of the liver. The other findings are very uncommon in early childhood. On occasion, the child may present with jaundice and acute hemolytic anemia..but this is much less common than liver disease and cirrhosis.

117. Answer: D

The correct answer is hypertrophic pyloric stenosis. Infants with pyloric stenosis generally have been vomiting for several days to weeks before the diagnosis is made. They chronically are losing gastric acid which results in a metabolic alkalosis. Hypokalemic metabolic alkalosis is the most common acid-base disturbance seen in these infants. All of the other conditions listed are associated with a metabolic acidosis except for aspirin toxicity which initially would result in a respiratory alkalosis.

118. Answer: A

The correct answer is diarrhea—which is usually not seen in this disorder. The disorder is due to a deficiency in the liver of fructose-1-phosphate aldolase, which results in impaired metabolism of dietary fructose. If fructose is eaten, this results in vomiting, hepatomegaly, jaundice, hypoglycemia, lethargy, coma and eventually death. A fructose-free diet will result in resolution of symptoms.

119. Answer: A

The correct answer is homocystinuria. This is an autosomal recessive disorder of amino acid metabolism in which there is a defect in the activity of cystathionine synthetase, the enzyme that catalyzes the metabolism of homocystine and serine to cystathionine.

120. Answer: B

The correct answer is Niemann-Pick (Type A) disease. This is one of the inborn errors of metabolism known as the sphingolipidoses. These disorders are characterized by accumulation of lipids in the central nervous system or the liver and spleen. Of these, Niemann-Pick is the only one to affect the liver and spleen. The cherry red spot is seen in about 30% of patients. Tay-Sachs disease presents very similarly except there is no hepatosplenomegaly. Remember that little tidbit—it maybe the only thing you have to separate the two! Gaucher's disease does not have the cherry red spot and neither does globoid-cell leukodystrophy or Biotin deficiency.

121. Answer: A

The correct answer is seizures. Seizures are not a part of this syndrome. Early on, the infants don't feed well but they make up for it in childhood and develop excessive appetites and obesity. The obesity accentuates the micropenis—ok, don't get mad at me for putting this in—it is in 2 textbooks of Pediatrics!! The hypotonia lessens with age.

122. Answer: E

The correct answer is metabolic alkalosis. Malignant hyperthermia is most frequently transmitted as an autosomal dominant disorder. Metabolic acidosis is seen, not metabolic alkalosis. Anesthetic agents like halothane or succinylcholine trigger attacks. CPK is markedly elevated during the attacks.

123. Answer: C

The correct "incorrect" answer is sepsis due to *Arcanobacterium*. They *are* at risk from sepsis but from encapsulated organisms like *Streptococcus pneumoniae, Haemophilus influenzae,* or *Neisseria meningococcus*. All of the other findings are seen with the congenital absence of the spleen.

124. Answer: A

The correct answer is Tay-Sachs disease. The findings of a cherry red spot on the macula should narrow it down to Tay-Sachs or Niemann-Pick disease. The lack of hepatosplenomegaly supports Tay-Sachs as the correct diagnosis.

125. Answer: C

The correct answer is Fabry's disease. Note Fabry's is an X-Linked recessive disorder—this is a GIRL! Plus Fabry's has little or no central nervous system findings.

126. Answer: C

The correct answer is DiGeorge's syndrome. There is an abnormality of development of the structures arising from the third and fourth pharyngeal pouches. There is absence of the thymus and the parathyroid glands, with resultant immunodeficiency and hypocalcemia. Chronic infections are common with bacterial, viral, and fungal organisms. Infants with severe combined immunodeficiency do not have ear abnormalities or hypocalcemia. Infants with renal failure, idiopathic hypoparathyroidism or autoimmune disease would not be expected to have an absent thymus on CXR.

127. Answer: B

The correct answer is Trisomy 18 (Edward's syndrome). Most of these babies die in early infancy. They have "abnormal fisting" with their index finger overlying the third finger. They usually have a VSD or PDA. Their face is round with a narrow forehead, frontal bossing, hypertelorism, micrognathia, and antimongoloid palpebral fissures.

128. Answer: C

The correct answer is 45, XO or Turner's syndrome. The older child will present with short stature, lack of development of sexual characteristics, primary amenorrhea, webbing of the neck, cubitus valgus, and short 4th metacarpals. They have ovarian dysgenesis. Coarctation is classically seen as are bicuspid aortic valves.

129. Answer: A

The correct answer is Trisomy 13 (Patau's syndrome). This syndrome classically has holoprosencephaly, cleft lip and palate, and severe mental retardation. Remember what holoprosencephaly is? I always have to remind myself—it is incomplete development of the forebrain— it is often associated with absence of the corpus callosum and fusion of the frontal lobes as well as a single ventricle. Eye findings are common as are cardiac findings. Scalp defects are common and may be helpful in diagnosis.

130. Answer: D

The correct answer is 5p- deletion (cri du chat syndrome). The characteristic cry, and also the dead-ringer for this question, goes away by 1 to 2 years of age. The cry is high pitched and distinctive. It is because of a small, narrow, hypoplastic larynx!

131. Answer: B

The correct answer is Trisomy 21 (Down's syndrome). This is rather common, occurring in 1/770 live births. Less than 5% will have a translocation rather than an extra (47) chromosome. Simian creases of the palm, an increased distance between the 1st and 2nd toes, upward slanting palpebral fissures, epicanthal folds, flat nasal bridge, and flat occiput are some of the physical findings seen. Brushfield's spots are tiny white spots that form a ring in the mid-zone of the iris. These are present in up to 25% of normal folk, especially those with blue eyes.

132. Answer: C

The answer is: Angelman syndrome (also known as Happy Puppet syndrome). The typical phenotype includes abnormal puppet-like gait and movements, seizures, significant motor delays, poor speech development, paroxysmal laughter, and tongue thrusting. Sixty-five percent have blond hair and 88% have blue eyes. They can also have maxillary hypoplasia and deep-set eyes. Angelman syndrome is most commonly caused by deletion of sequences on 15q11 from the maternal homologue.

133. Answer: A

The answer is variable phenotypic expression depending on the parent of origin of the deleted chromosome. An example is deletion of chromosome 15q11-13. Paternal deletion results in the patient having Prader-Willi syndrome, whereas with maternal deletion, the result is Angelman syndrome. This suggests that identical genes possess dissimilar function depending on whether they are passed from the mother or father.

134. Answer: E

The answer is karyotype. This patient demonstrates the characteristics of Klinefelter syndrome including hypogonadism, dull mentality, and/or behavioral problems. The diagnosis is rarely made prior to puberty due to the lack of clinical manifestations in childhood. Although the I.Q. range is quite variable (from well below average to some above average), the mean I.Q. is between 85-90. They usually exhibit behavioral problems ranging from shyness and immaturity to aggressiveness. They tend to be tall and slim with long legs and a mean height at the 75th percentile. Once they hit puberty, their testes remain small with low testosterone, elevated gonadotropins, sparse facial hair, azoospermia and infertility. Eighty percent of adults have gynecomastia. The diagnosis is made by karyotype which shows 47 XXY. Treatment is replacement therapy with a long-acting testosterone.

135. Answer: B

The answer is: Crouzon syndrome. Crouzon syndrome is caused by a mutation to chromosome 10q25-q26 and has an autosomal dominant transmission. The typical features include shallow orbits causing proptosis, premature craniosynostosis, and maxillary hypoplasia. Patients can also exhibit hypertelorism, frontal bossing, conductive hearing loss, poor visual acuity, optic atrophy, and nystagmus. Surgical procedures for more normal brain development are only indicated for increased intracranial pressure. Otherwise surgery is for cosmetic purposes. There are also surgical procedures for facial bone reconstruction.

136. Answer: A

The answer is bring him in right away for evaluation and lab tests. The number one complication of varicella is bacterial superinfection of the lesions. Any patient who continues to run fever 5 days into the illness (he is at day 6 now) needs to be re-evaluated with CBC and blood cultures.

137. Answer: D

The correct answer is Rabies Immune Globulin (1/2 into the wound and ½ IM in separate site from vaccine) and Rabies Vaccine IM in the deltoid region. Obviously she needs the preventative therapy, right? The key is knowing if it is IM or SQ. There is an SQ version of this vaccine—BUT it is only for Pre-exposure prophylaxis—used for veterinarians or those working with potentially Rabid Animals (or Boxers who bite?). The Deltoid is the preferred region for the vaccine. The old vaccine used to be given in the abdominal area.

138. Answer: C

The correct answer is Deborah, all other attendees, and all adults working in the daycare should receive rifampin prophylaxis. Once 2 cases are confirmed in a daycare setting, then all children as well as adults working in the center should receive prophylaxis with rifampin. This is to "break the cycle" and eliminate *H. influenzae* carriage in the nasal pharynx. Even completely immunized children can still carry the organism in their nose as well as have a small risk of acute infection.

139. Answer: E

The correct answer is Wendy and all children as well as adult workers who have had close contact with the infected index case should be prophylaxed with appropriate antibiotics. With *Neisseria meningitides* infection, one case in a day care warrants prophylaxis for those in close contact with the index case. The risk of invasive disease increases nearly 400-500 fold for those who are in close intimate contact with an index case. Remember with *H. influenzae,* 2 cases are the "cut-off", as opposed to meningococcus—which only requires 1 case.

140. Answer: D

The correct answer is once the rash appears, the infection is generally not infectious—he may return to school now. If you had diagnosed the infection somehow before the rash appeared, you would have recommended—nothing. The risk of a severe outcome in a pregnant teacher is less than 1%. Also, nearly 20% of infections are asymptomatic. Pregnant school teachers are not at any increased risk for fetal infection as compared to the general population.

141. Answer: C

The correct answer is the 6th day after onset of the rash or sooner if all lesions are dried and crusted. The 6th day is chosen generally because viral loads are markedly decreased by this day. Some children will crust over earlier and this indicates the infection has also abated.

142. Answer: C

The correct answer is as long as the lesion is kept covered by her clothes she may return to work now. Lesions that can be covered pose little risk—as transmission in zoster occurs via direct contact with fluid from the lesions.

143. Answer: E

The correct answer is all of the choices are possible routes of infection.
This was a pretty easy one, right? Just figured you needed a break for a second before answering a question about *Trypanosoma brucei gambiense* infection (oh yea..this causes African sleeping sickness).

144. Answer: A

The correct answer is *Mycoplasma pneumoniae*. For all of the other organisms listed, the use of treatment or prophylaxis will prevent spread of the infection. For *Mycoplasma*, treatment does not appear to limit spread of this infection nor does it eradicate the organism.

145. Answer: C

The correct answer is private room, negative air-pressure ventilation, masks at all times, standard precautions. Measles is spread via the air-borne route. As such, all of the requirements listed are necessary. Remember, negative-pressure keeps the "infected air" IN and prevents spread to the rest of the corridor on the hallway. Standard precautions are implemented for "ALL" patients regardless of what infection they have.

146. Answer: A

The correct answer is diphtheria. All of the other infections require "contact" isolation only. Droplet transmission precautions would include a private room and use of a mask if within 3 feet of patient. This is true for infections such as invasive *H. influenzae*, *N. meningitides*, Pertussis, Streptoccocal infections, Adenovirus, Influenza, mumps, parvovirus B 19, and rubella. Measles, varicella, and tuberculosis require "airborne" precautions—meaning mask at ALL times.

147. Answer: D

The correct answer is clean the wound and start amoxicillin-clavulanate. A bite wound to the hand or foot is usually impetus to start antimicrobial therapy. The agent of choice is amoxicillin-clavulanate— mainly due to risk of *Staphylococcus aureus*, various streptococci, *Pasteurella multocida*, anaerobes, and *Capnocytophaga canimorsus* (mainly in dogs). If he was penicillin allergic, the drug of choice would have been an extended spectrum cephalosporin or trimethoprim-sulfamethoxazole PLUS clindamycin.

148. Answer: A

The correct answer is start amoxicillin-clavulanate. The most common organisms with human bite wounds are various Streptococci, *Staphylococcus aureus*, *Eikenella corrodens*, and anaerobes. The best choice is amoxicillin-clavulanate. Note, if he had been penicillin allergic then trimethoprim-sulfamethoxazole PLUS clindamycin would have been an alternative.

149. Answer: D

The correct answer is grasp with a fine tweezer close to the skin and remove by gently pulling the tick straight out without twisting motions. All of the other methods are likely to irate the tick more—which will result in it regurgitating, defecating, or urinating into the bite would—thus increasing the risk of release of infectious organisms. (DISGUSTING ISN'T IT—the idea of a tick defecating in your bite wound)!

150. Answer: A

The correct answer is *Actinomyces israelii*. The key here is if you see the words "sulfur" granules in a mouth abscess or other abscess (thoracic, tonsillar, appendix/cecum) go for Actinomyces!! It also can occur with and is also associated with IUD use in an adolescent. Treatment is with intravenous penicillin G or ampicillin for 4-6 weeks; followed with oral therapy for 6-12 MONTHS!! Yes, it is a serious infection. Don't miss this easy question on the Boards—sulfur granules=Actinomyces!!

151. Answer: D

The correct answer is adenovirus. Think of this in an "epidemic" involving a swimming pool—particularly if kids are sharing towels, etc. Another thing to think about with this organism is hemorrhagic cystitis—it is really rare but the Boards will ask about it for some crazy reason. Adenovirus can also cause pharyngitis, gastroenteritis, pneumonia and croup. The other question they will ask about is a Peds resident who has adenoviral conjunctivitis—can they work? NO. They must be removed from patient care duties until the illness has resolved.

152. Answer: D

The correct answer is an arbovirus. She most likely had one of the arboviruses endemic for her region of the United States. Most common arboviruses in outbreaks in the United States include St. Louis, Western Equine, and LaCrosse viruses. Most infections are actually asymptomatic. Mosquitoes are the vector and effective control of the infection in the area centers on the control of the mosquito population. There is no effective therapy for arboviruses. Recently, West-Nile virus has migrated to the United States. It is a prime time to be on the Peds Boards—look for a patient who lives in the New York, Louisiana or Florida area; Look for non-specific symptoms and some comment about mosquitoes and summertime. Also, suspect this infection if they say a "bunch of birds" have died in the area.

153. Answer: B

The correct answer is parvovirus B-19. Buster, the child, has the classic "5th's disease" with slapped cheeks and a serpiginous rash that worsens with heat or sun exposure. She has the classic adult manifestation with arthralgias and frank arthritis. This is yet another manifestation of this virus--don't forget this virus causes aplastic anemia especially in AIDS or sickle cell patients. Human herpesvirus 6 causes Roseola in kids and is responsible for pneumonia, meningitis, etc. in immunocompromised adults. She doesn't have Lyme disease even though you may have taken the bait with her being from New Lyme, Connecticut (Do you really think I would make it that obvious??). Remember <u>she's</u> had no fever, no rash. If she had "frank" arthritis with <u>effusion</u> I'd suspect it more likely. Disseminated gonorrhea in this lady and her child?? That would involve issues that I don't want to get into plus, his rash is not classic for gonorrhea and she has no rash and no evidence of disseminated pustules.

154. Answer: D

The correct answer is intravenous penicillin G or Ampicillin. This unfortunate child has bacteremia with Listeria, a gram-positive diphtheroid-like organism. Think of this organism—in the neonate less than 2 months, in pregnancy, or someone who eats a lot of goat or imported cheeses, particularly from Mexico. Penicillin or Ampicillin is the only thing that will get it reliably. If she is penicillin allergic you could use trimethoprim/sulfamethoxazole—but you'd be worried about the trimethoprim/sulfamethoxazole too with her pregnancy. Normally if you hear about a diphtheroid-like organism you suspect contamination—however in someone immunocompromised or semi-immunocompromised (like neonates or pregnancy) don't ignore it until you are sure it comes back as something unimportant.

155. Answer: B

The correct answer is to treat again with metronidazole. With *C. difficile* diarrhea it is expected that up to 1/3 of patients may relapse no matter what therapy you use. Therefore repeat therapy with metronidazole is reasonable. Oral vancomycin costs about $300 and is difficult to find. Clindamycin is not an appropriate choice—remember on a dose-by-dose basis clindamycin causes *C. difficile* more often than any other antibiotic. BUT, if they ask you which antibiotics cause *C. difficile* diarrhea, the most likely are the beta-lactams—because they are used a lot more than other antibiotics. So this is still confusing?? Look at it this way. Which antibiotic (clindamycin or cephalosporin) is more likely to induce *C. difficile* diarrhea in a single patient? The answer is clindamycin.
Which antibiotic, nationwide, more commonly causes *C. difficile* diarrhea: cephalosporin. Got it now?

156. Answer: B

The answer is: incision & drainage followed by antibiotics. This patient has a pilonidal abscess. Antibiotics alone are ineffective at clearing the bacteria of a soft tissue abscess. This requires incision & drainage. After drainage and irrigation, the cavity should be packed with packing gauze and covered with gauze pads. Follow-up wound check should be in 24-48 hours for packing removal and possible repacking.

157. Answer: A

The correct answer is *Staphylococcus aureus*. This organism is responsible for over 90% of these infections. Empiric antibiotic coverage should include an anti-staphylococcal antibiotic.

158. Answer: E

The correct answer is intestinal obstruction. All of the other items listed are classic presentations for CMV infection that has caused morbidity in a neonate. Luckily, most CMV infections are asymptomatic!

159. Answer: C

The correct answer is the mortality is still near 20% with a significant risk of neurologic sequelae in the survivors. The prognosis is still poor for neonates with bacterial meningitis.

160. Answer: A

The correct answer is meningitis. "Late-onset" presents as meningitis; early-onset presents as sepsis and pneumonia.

161. Answer: E

The correct answer is gram stain of the exudate. This is simple and easy (In other words—THIS IS WHAT THE BOARDS LIKE ☺). A gram stain that shows gram negative diplococci will pretty much nail your diagnosis for you! You still would get a culture to confirm but with that information you would definitely treat the child. Silver nitrate prophylaxis is not 100%--so even if you personally put in the silver nitrate and spread it everywhere—it is still possible the kid is infected. The other thing the ABP does NOT like is treating something infectious—without getting appropriate cultures.

162. Answer: B

The correct answer is most newborn infants are susceptible to pertussis. There is little transplacental protection with pertussis. This is a growing problem. Be on the look out on the exam for a coughing infant with a coughing parent, grandparent, or older sibling!!

163. Answer: A

The correct answer is maternal antibodies are protective. Neonatal tetanus is rare in the United States. If the baby is born in a hospital in sterile conditions then it is very unlikely to get tetanus—even if the mother is unimmunized, or is an intravenous drug user. Also, hypocalcemia causes the symptoms of tetanus but does not predispose the infant to tetanus. Look for it on the exam in a "refugee" from another country who is an illegal immigrant here and has the baby at home.

164. Answer: A

The correct answer is doxycycline 100 mg bid x 21 days. She has classic lyme arthritis. She lives in an endemic area and she had a classic erythema migrans 5 months ago. She does not have any other signs of gonorrhea (like disseminated skin lesions). Also with gonorrhea the joint manifestations are usually migratory. In no circumstances would you give her ciprofloxacin anyway—she is less than 18 years of age. You were thinking this possibly could be parvovirus B19 but I helped you out by not giving any choices here appropriate for that.

165. Answer: A

The correct answer is *Chlamydia pneumoniae*. The constellation of symptoms: chronic non-productive cough, low-grade fever, hyperemic sore throat, hoarseness fit this infection. *C. psittaci* is a concern BUT he has no hepatosplenomegaly. Expect them to give you splenomegaly with this infection. A combination of pneumonia with splenomegaly: think *C. psittaci* or *Coxiella burnetii*!! *Coxiella* I'd also think about if they said he delivered cows or some livestock or more recently CATS have been implicated with this infection—but you have to have contact with placentas usually for this. *S. pneumoniae* is unlikely to produce this prolonged gradual infection and the patchy infiltrate goes against it somewhat. Plus they kept saying he had no chills—if you see "chills" and "rusty sputum" think of *S. pneumoniae*.

166. Answer: D

The correct answer is intravenous penicillin G or Ampicillin. This baby has bacteremia with Listeria, a gram-positive diphtheroid-like organism. Think of this organism in a baby less than 2 months of age or an adolescent who is pregnant or someone who eats a lot of goat or imported cheeses, particularly from Mexico. Penicillin or Ampicillin is the only thing that will get it reliably. If she is penicillin allergic you could use trimethoprim/sulfamethoxazole. Normally if you hear about a diphtheroid-like organism you suspect contamination—however in babies or the immunocompromised or semi-immunocompromised (like pregnancy) don't ignore it until you are sure it comes back as something unimportant.

167. Answer: A

The correct "incorrect" answer is *Salmonella*. Remember with Salmonella that treatment in "normal" hosts prolongs the time of active shedding. Therefore with Salmonella you do not treat with antibiotics in a "normal" host.

168. Answer: D

The correct answer is ceftriaxone and vancomycin. She has pneumococcal meningitis. Realize that in many parts of the United States up to 30% of pneumococci are resistant to penicillin and up to 10% are resistant to the 3rd generation cephalosporins. Know that Vancomycin and ceftriaxone are appropriate for presumed pneumococcal meningitis until the sensitivities are known. Another option is ceftriaxone and rifampin. Her prior antibiotic usage increases her risk of having a resistant organism. Ceftazidime is a poor choice as it has diminished gram-positive activity compared to ceftriaxone and cefotaxime. Penicillin alone would be a poor choice because of the high resistant rates. Now, if they tell you the pneumococcus is sensitive to penicillin then that would be the correct choice!

169. Answer: A

The correct answer is Herpes simplex meningoencephalitis. The key here is the "bizarre behavior" and the findings on MRI of temporal lobe involvement. To help you diagnose this, a PCR for Herpes simplex virus DNA could be helpful on the CSF. CSF cultures for herpes are rarely positive except in the severely immunocompromised or in neonates. He certainly is at risk for syphilis but the CSF findings don't support it nor does the MRI. You would though order a CSF VDRL on this kid just because he is at high risk based on his past history. *Bartonella henselae* is the etiology for Cat Scratch disease and does cause significant CNS disease in children on occasion-usually it will present with seizures. Seizures are also very common with Herpes encephalitis too. We have no indication he has varicella and this does not look like bacterial meningitis with the normal protein and glucose.

170. Answer: B

The correct answer is Sucralfate. This agent will substantially interfere with the absorption of the oral drug resulting in sub-therapeutic serum and urine levels. Other agents to avoid that also will do this include antacids that contain magnesium, aluminum, or calcium. Theophylline is another agent to avoid as concurrent ciprofloxacin will cause increases in theophylline levels and possible theophylline toxicity. I know, the quinolones are never used in pediatrics—however, be prepared..studies will be coming out soon that many feel will finally allow quinolone usage for the pediatric population. Plus, they are commonly used in Cystic Fibrosis patients—so you need to know a little about the quinolones for the ABP!

171. Answer: C

The correct answer is *Pseudomonas aeruginosa*. This is the most common cause of acute otitis externa in patients with diabetes. Note, this guy needs admission and needs to be treated with intravenous antibiotics that cover Pseudomonas well. Choices would include piperacillin/tazobactam or ceftazidime. The other choices can cause otitis externa but are less common especially in diabetics. Oh, the *Streptococcus diabeticus* was something I just made up—sorry, it is very near my vacation when I'm writing this—I thought I might as well make your day fun too.

172. Answer: C

The correct answer is penicillin G 3 million units intravenously q 4 hours. This patient has neurosyphilis. But, you say—the CSF VDRL was negative. How can she have neurosyphilis? Because I say so that's why. Actually, remember that the CSF VDRL is very SPECIFIC (meaning that if it is positive it means they truly have neurosyphilis) but it is not very SENSITIVE (only about ½ of patients with documented neurosyphilis will have a positive CSF VDRL!!). So you knew she had syphilis right? The serum VDRL and FTA-ABS were both positive. If you do an LP on someone with neurologic findings and they have a positive RPR or VDRL on their serum that is relatively high you are going to have to consider that they might have neurosyphilis. She has meningitis by definition with 50 WBCs in her CSF. And she has an elevated abnormal protein in the CSF. Both go along with neurosyphilis. So, she's got neurosyphilis. And the poor girl also has AIDS too which she didn't know she had before coming to see you.

Note: Look also for syphilis in a young person with hearing loss or alopecia!!!!! Always look for syphilis in them!

173. Answer: A

The correct answer is *Pseudomonas aeruginosa*. Note, he is only 5 days out from his transplant. The most common organisms to cause problems this early are hospital-acquired infections particularly with gram-negatives like *Pseudomonas*. Note CMV and *Pneumocystis* are likely in 1-4 months out. *Cryptococcus* is a problem more often 4 or more months out. *Legionella* really doesn't have much more increased incidence unless there was something wrong with the processing of water in the hospital.

174. Answer: B

The correct answer is *Bartonella henselae*. This patient has Cat Scratch Fever or disease. Who wrote the song Cat Scratch Fever? That's right Ted Nugent. Note, commonly you'll see patients present with axillary nodes and scratches on the hand—that is just too dang easy. But know that a classic conjunctivitis pre-auricular node syndrome is Cat Scratch disease. This is not Lyme disease. This is not Herpes. This is really not likely to be MRSA. And the poor turtle here is innocent so *Aeromonas* is not a problem either. Remember for the Boards: Common things are common; rare things are rare. What causes lymph node swelling in a child exposed to animals (particularly kittens) that does not respond to anti-Staph drugs?? Most common thing is going to be Cat Scratch.

175. Answer: A

The correct answer is Cytomegalovirus retinitis. CMV retinitis is the most common eye disorder to occur in adolescent and adult patients with CD4 counts below 50. Patients will frequently initially complain of floaters and gradually they will lose vision. This patient has classic findings on ophthalmologic examination: Attenuation of vessels in the area affected by retinitis. Retinal lesions will occur as two possible presentations. In the posterior type, large areas of thick white infiltrate are accompanied by retinal hemorrhage, with a distribution along retinal vessels. The peripheral type demonstrates granular retinitis with satellite lesions and less hemorrhage. Behind the advancing border is necrotic retina. Treatment is with intravenous ganciclovir, foscarnet or both. Also it is important to get her HIV under better control and with better anti-HIV therapy raise her CD4. This would be very helpful in controlling her disease.

176. Answer: C

The correct answer is Methicillin-resistant *Staphylococcus epidermidis*. This is a straightforward knowledge question. Remember with prosthetic valve endocarditis that occurs within the first 2 months, Methicillin-resistant *Staphylococcus epidermidis* (MRSE) is the most common organism. It also is the most common after 2 months—so that one is easy to remember. Prosthetic valve endocarditis: MRSE. Treatment is with Vancomycin + rifampin + gentamicin initially. For Native valve endocarditis it gets a little more confusing.

For adolescents and young adults divide it this way:

For the Non-addict: Divide it into Acute (Usually no-previously known valve problem, Janeway lesions) vs. Subacute (usually a previous valvular abnormality, Osler nodes, Roth spots). For acute--think of *Staphylococcus aureus*. For subacute--think of the viridans group of Streptococci (mouth strep too).

For the addict, also divide into acute and non-acute: Acute will be *S. aureus* or *Pseudomonas*. For the subacute, think *Enterococcus*, Viridans type of Strep or Fungi like *Candida*. (Particularly for right sided).

For the culture-negative; non-addict think of HACEK, fungal, and weird things like Q-fever or *Chlamydia psittaci*.

For the child, think of the same organisms as the non-addict adult—usually a *Streptococcus* of the viridans group (50%) or *Enterococcus* (depending on age) or *Streptococcus pneumoniae*. *Staphylococcus aureus* is also fairly common in this age group.

177. Answer: E

The correct answer is assay for acute and convalescent titers. This patient has (drum roll please) Tularemia. To diagnose Tularemia which is due to *Francisella tularensis* you usually will do acute and convalescent serum titers. You do NOT want to biopsy or aspirate a lymph node with tularemia. You are putting yourself and the lab at risk for aerosolization of the organism. Febrile agglutinins are WORTHLESS. CAN I SAY IT STRONGER? NEVER EVER ORDER febrile agglutinins on anybody on the ABP!!!!!!!! Treatment of this boy would be with IM streptomycin, IV gentamicin or oral doxycycline. He doesn't appear to be that ill so oral doxycycline might be worth a trial. There is a higher risk of relapse with oral doxycycline though.

178. Answer: B

The correct answer is Ehrlichiosis. This patient has fever and non-specific symptoms. He has splenomegaly. He has pancytopenia with elevated liver transaminases. This picture goes with Ehrlichiosis. For tularemia, you would expect lymphadenopathy and not expect to find a pancytopenia. Histoplasma and Blasto would be unusual to present in this fashion. This also is not a presentation for Lyme disease.

179. Answer: C

The correct answer is *Neisseria gonorrhoeae*. Ms. Smith has the classic findings of disseminated gonorrhea. Note, if she was having her menses that would have been even more indicative of this type of infection.

Remember that females are more likely to have this than males. It is unlikely that you will grow the organism from the blood but possibly from the genitourinary tract. The other thing to remember is that ceftriaxone is the treatment of choice because of the resistance problem with penicillin in the United States. None of the other choices would fit this picture except for possibly *Streptococcus pyogenes* but endocarditis would have to be in the differential and she has no evidence of this from the history—although we know she lied about her sexual history. Most of the time on the Board's people tell the truth—except when it is a teenager and you are discussing sex or drugs (or rock and roll). On the Boards, they will frequently tell you their true sexual history---but if they don't—it is just like real life and they LIE, LIE, LIE about it!

180. Answer: D

The correct answer is to call for an immediate ENT or Anesthesia consultation and start ceftriaxone now. This patient has acute epiglottitis. The usual organisms are *Haemophilus influenzae* and more recently *Streptococcus pyogenes*. Classically this was a disease of childhood but with *H. influenzae* immunization this disease has decreased markedly in incidence. The other antibiotic choices are not good choices for *H. influenzae*. The choice of initially culturing the throat is definitely a no-no. You should do as little as possible in manipulation of the oropharynx. Frequently you don't even want to look in the mouth if it will upset the patient. That is why immediate ENT or anesthesia back up is needed for protection of the patient's airway.

181. Answer: D

The correct answer is HIV ELISA. Patients with HIV infection have an increased risk of having recurrent infections with Salmonella particularly *S. typhimurium*. KNOW THIS: If someone has recurrent bacteremias with *Salmonella typhimurium* or *Streptococcus pneumoniae* think about HIV! The other choices are much less likely to be helpful in this patient. Also be aware that complement deficiency can predispose to these infections too; as well as Sickle Cell patients and others without functional spleens.

182. Answer: A

The correct answer is *Clostridium tetani*. This kid has TETANUS!! Look for it in unimmunized adults or babies born at home to unimmunized mothers (On exams—but, in real life, this RARELY occurs in the US—except with the elderly). Classically, older patients will present with "lockjaw" and then progress to have the other symptoms. The weird opisthotonic posturing described is classic for tetanus. Note, that the only other thing that will do this is strychnine poisoning. Dystonic reactions to drugs can also look like this, but remember that usually this involves LATERAL HEAD TURNING which is very rare in tetanus. Dental infections may produce trismus but do not cause the other manifestations of tetanus. Treatment is well laid out in many texts: always protect the airway, administer diphenhydramine to be sure you are not dealing with a dystonic reaction; then proceed to giving a benzodiazepine to control spasms and decrease rigidity. Treatment consists of administering Human tetanus immunoglobulin and immunization with Td (tetanus toxoid). Metronidazole is also given for 7-10 days. The course can be quite prolonged and require 6-8 weeks of intense rehabilitative therapy. Patients will receive 3 Td doses over the period of 8 weeks—hopefully he'll accept therapy and see the benefit of immunizations!

183. Answer: D

The correct answer is begin Combivir (Zidovudine/lamivudine) and nevirapine. She most likely has HIV-related immune thrombocytopenia—this is very COMMON in HIV infected individuals. Treatment with combination therapy has shown to be most effective (especially those using Zidovudine). Steroids would be contraindicated in this immunocompromised patient and we have no evidence that parvovirus B-19 might be involved with a severe anemia so use of IVIG is also not warranted. She is not actively bleeding and her platelet count is above 20,000 so there is no need to transfuse her with platelets at this time. If you see pancytopenia; think of an opportunistic disease.

184. Answer: C

The correct answer is *Yersinia enterocolitica*. I don't know if they will ask about this or not—but just in case, I threw this question in. There has been a lot of literature about transfusion related infections—most commonly they are due to *Pseudomonas* BUT recently there have been well documented cases due to *Yersinia enterocolitica*. This organism grows in high concentrations in stored packed red cells because of contamination by an asymptomatic donor with bacteremia. The organism grows well at the temperature blood is stored and grows really well in the presence of iron and dextran! This may be too esoteric for the general Peds Boards but I just have a feeling they might have something about this as one of their "toughie" questions. Now you won't miss it.

185. Answer: C

The correct answer is hepatitis B vaccine and hepatitis B immune globulin. The mother is most likely a carrier with hepatitis B infection. She can pass this to her newborn infant at delivery and therefore the child should receive both hepatitis B immune globulin as well as vaccine within the first 12 hours of birth! They should be given in two separate sites also. This is true for any instance in which you are giving an "immune globulin" type product and the vaccine concurrently. Otherwise the immune globulin will "bind-up" the vaccine and prevent an immunologic response from occurring in the recipient of the vaccine. Note this scenario would also work for someone who was exposed to a person with Hepatitis B—as with a sexual exposure or a needlestick exposure. Note also that if the exposed person has received vaccine and is known immune; you don't have to do anything as that is the purpose of the vaccine—it will protect the exposed person.

186. Answer: A

The correct answer is *Mycobacterium marinum*. Think about this organism in someone who is around water and marine organisms. For humans, the most common method of getting this is minor trauma. Particularly contact with fish spines or crustaceans. The infection takes awhile to incubate usually 2-3 weeks and obviously will not respond to routine antibiotics. Sporotrichosis, chromomycosis, and Blastomycosis can also all present like this—but nothing in the history helps us think about these. *Vibrio vulnificus* is also associated with water BUT you would expect to see BULLOUS skin lesions and it is usually seen in someone with liver disease particularly adult alcoholics. If the dad or mom owns fish tanks and the kids are sticking their hands down in the tanks a lot trying to grab at the fish—think of this organism too.

Oh yeah, Bartonella crustacea does not exist (yet) and there is no such thing as Crab Scratch fever—until a new Ted Nugent decides to write that one.

187. Answer: E

The correct answer is Herpes simplex virus. Even though this boy has been in an area with possible tularemia it is very unlikely to present in this fashion. He has not been in an endemic area for Lyme disease (*Borrelia burgdorferi*). Listeria and Streptococcus are much less likely based on his CSF findings. The protein and glucose are normal which indicates more likely a viral etiology. Also, his confusion—indicates an encephalitis is also occurring, which more commonly occurs with Herpes infection than with any of the other organisms listed.

188. Answer: D

The correct answer is Enterotoxigenic *Escherichia coli*. She has "Montezuma's" revenge. This is usually a non-bloody diarrhea that resolves without treatment. Eating leafy vegetables or uncooked foods will expose travelers to this organism. Additionally, ice and water are another common source as travelers mistakenly think that ice is protective. Also, a few people feel like the alcohol in a mixed drink will kill the bacteria—sorry it doesn't work that way. The other bacteria listed would generally cause much longer symptoms and more extensive disease. Remember with *E. coli* 0157:H7 NOT to give antibiotics—this is new from several reports in the NEJM in recent years. Rotavirus is unlikely and you would expect it more often in a daycare setting or younger children.

189. Answer: D

The correct answer is *Staphylococcus aureus*. Note this is a toughie unless you put together everything. "Mucous membrane changes; hypotension; Rash; Renal involvement, Liver involvement, Hematologic involvement. What gives you hypotension with a rash and multi-organ involvement with a history of trauma?? Toxic Shock Syndrome!! And that is what this poor kid has. Change the dog bite to say a scratch from a piece of metal or a post-op patient after surgery. Now does it make more sense?? The dog bite may have tricked you, but remember he is NOT immunocompromised. This kid is a normal dude. Disseminated *Pasteurella* and *Eikenella* are really unusual and unlikely to give you this constellation of findings—Endocarditis yes—but multiorgan involvement no. *Bartonella henselae* (Cat Scratch) would not do this either. That leaves *Neisseria* and it is possible BUT the trauma history is what should have led you to *Staphylococcus*. I told you this one is hard..BUT when you get someone with multi-organ involvement and a RASH think of Toxic Shock syndrome—either due to *Staphylococcus* or *Streptococcus pyogenes*!!

190. Answer: A

The correct answer is False-positive HIV ELISA for HIV-1. She never should have been told she had HIV infection. False-positive HIV ELISAs are quite common; that is why we must wait for the Western blot results. Unfortunately, indeterminate Western blots are also seen occasionally. They generally are false-positive results and are positive in only 1 band that is tested. The other thing to note is that this patient is really at low-risk. When you test a low-risk population with a highly sensitive test you are likely to see a large number of false-positive test results. It was possible early on that this was early HIV-1 infection; however by 3 months and 6 months she should have developed more bands. Resolved HIV infection in adults has not been clinically described. HIV-2 infection would show up on the Western blot. The other choice, that this is a false-negative Western blot, is very unlikely at this point.

191. Answer: E

The correct answer is Papanicolaou smear, RPR, HIV counseling, GC and *Chlamydia* culturing. Note, that HSV culturing is not likely to be helpful. If she is asymptomatic you would not treat her even if she had positive cultures and it would not be causing her discharge. Culturing for *Gardnerella* is not cost-effective, is difficult to do, and likely would not yield meaningful results. *Candida* culturing is not going to be helpful. She likely is colonized and so even if you find the organism it doesn't necessarily mean that it is causing the problem. You must determine if she has gonorrhea or *Chlamydia*. Both are treatable diseases and it is important for her to know and for the public health officials in the community to be aware of either of these infections so that partner notification can occur.

192. Answer: A

The correct answer is No prophylaxis is indicated. Note, that urine is not on the list of body fluids to be worried about with transmission. Blood, semen, vaginal secretions, CSF, synovial, pleural, peritoneal, pericardial and amniotic fluid are considered "potentially infectious fluids". Let's say this was blood in a cup. Mr. Cerf would have exposure to blood of large volume to what would be considered "skin with integrity potentially compromised". The source patient's HIV viral load is really high so we would offer Mr. Cerf the three drug therapy listed of zidovudine, lamivudine, and indinavir for 4 weeks. No data exists (at least as of July 2002) on whether you should change therapy based on genotypes. Some authorities currently recommend considering it but for Board purposes they won't ask you this. Remember for large amounts of infectious fluid exposure with a high viral load to use 3 drug prophylaxis! For non-infectious fluid or fluid that is only in contact with "intact skin only" no prophylaxis is indicated.

193. Answer: C

The correct answer is further evaluation for depression and referral for counseling. Mark has classic signs of depression with change in sleeping and eating patterns and loss of interest in usual entertaining activities. EBV serology has been blamed for many things from Chronic fatigue to a persistent EBV syndrome. So far most medical literature does not support this agent as a culprit for these syndromes. He has a completely normal examination. You have no documentable symptoms except his fatigue and he has had major life complications in the past year. These patients can be very difficult to convince that depression could be at the root of their problem. Frequently it takes a combination of medication as well as an effective counselor to help these patients get back to a normal life. After starting Mark on an antidepressant and receiving counseling, he returned to his youthful healthy self; lost 30lbs in 6 months and is on the hockey team at school. Not all patients are success stories like this; but it should be remembered that a non-specific laboratory test if misinterpreted can frequently cause more harm than good!

194. Answer: B

The correct answer is trimethoprim/sulfamethoxazole. This patient with advanced HIV disease develops hyperkalemia while being treated for PCP. TMP/Sulfa can block tubular potassium secretion and severe hyperkalemia has been reported in AIDS patients receiving IV TMP/Sulfa for the treatment of PCP. Hyperkalemia has also been reported in elderly patients receiving oral TMP/Sulfa. Although adrenal insufficiency can cause hyperkalemia and does occur in patients with advanced HIV disease, it would be unlikely in this patient because he received steroids (Solu-Medrol).

195. Answer: E

The correct answer is no therapy at this time. This patient is asymptomatic but has a positive urine culture for a frequently drug-resistant organism. Most chronically catheterized patients will have positive urine cultures. Treatment should only occur if the patient has a symptomatic infection. This patient is asymptomatic including a normal WBC. Attempted treatment would likely lead to a more drug-resistant organism without offering benefit to the patient

196. Answer: A

The correct answer is serum antibody test. He most likely has extra-intestinal amebiasis with liver involvement. Stool for ova and parasites are usually negative at this stage of disease and the liver aspirate is unlikely to show organisms. The treatment is metronidazole followed by a luminal amebicide.

197. Answer: D

The correct answer is *Naegleria fowleri* meningoencephalitis. This is VERY rare but occasionally shows up on the Boards. Think of this in an adolescent who is a country kid who swims in cow ponds or other areas where livestock are likely to share the swimming area. Unfortunately, this illness is almost always fatal. Treatment can be tried with Amphotericin B. Sometimes you can add miconazole or rifampin in combination.

198. Answer: B

The correct answer is *Acanthamoeba species*. This is a weird infection—but think about it in contact lens users—particularly if their "hygiene" may or may not be pristine. This is a difficult infection to treat and requires the help of an ophthalmologist. Just remember—if someone in the question is wearing contact lenses and gets an infection think about this weird organism!!

199. Answer: E

The correct answer is thick and thin smears of blood. This patient has probable Babesiosis due to *Babesia microti*—an intraerythrocytic protozoa. This is essentially the U.S. version of malaria. It is particularly a problem in those without spleens like William here. Treatment with clindamycin and quinine for 7 days is appropriate in someone severely ill like this patient. Most cases are likely asymptomatic. Serologic tests are available from the Centers for Disease Control and Prevention and some local State labs. A PCR is under investigation.

200. Answer: A

The correct answer is continue to search for other organisms like *Giardia* or *Cryptosporidium*. *Blastocystis hominis* is found commonly in as often as 20% of stool samples. The asymptomatic carrier state is quite common. However, if this organism is found it should warrant a search for other pathogens—particularly *Giardia* and *Cryptosporidium*. Some believe that in a "normal" host, this organism does not cause any infection—others feel it is true pathogen, especially in the immunocompromised. In any case, it is prudent to look for other causes of infection besides this organism.

201. Answer: D

The correct answer is KOH of the exudates. He most likely has blastomycosis. This is a relatively common infection in Arkansas, Missouri, the Chicago area, and Wisconsin—at least think about it if they present a kid from these areas with a complaint of pneumonia and draining skin lesions. Disseminated disease can spread to the brain, bone, liver, and kidney.

202. Answer: B

The correct answer is itraconazole and its metabolites are below therapeutic levels. The problem with itraconazole (and more so with ketoconazole) is that an ACID-stomach environment is helpful for absorption. When the patient was placed on ranitidine with his itraconazole the itraconazole was likely not absorbed. Therefore he has sub-therapeutic levels of itraconazole. It is very unlikely that he has cryptococcus now. Itraconazole-resistant Histoplasma is likely exceedingly rare. *Candida krusei* is unlikely also. Think about this: if a patient is on FLUCONAZOLE—that is when infections associated with *Candida krusei* will appear on Boards and the real world. Yeast that grows in a blood culture or seen on peripheral smear should NEVER be considered a contaminant.

203. Answer: A

The correct answer is azithromycin weekly. Of the choices listed, only the azithromycin weekly is currently approved for prophylaxis. Clarithromycin could be used but he would have to use it daily. Rifampin is not approved for MAI prophylaxis. Rifabutin and clarithromycin would be used for treatment not prophylaxis. The choice of "Nothing" is not correct, as he really is becoming high risk for MAI infection.

204. Answer: B

The correct answer is change the catheter site; add amphotericin B. She has infection with *Candida krusei* which is almost always resistant to fluconazole. Recent literature supports removal and replacement of a central venous catheter if cultures are positive for a *Candida sp.* or other fungemia. NEVER NEVER NEVER consider a *Candida* blood culture result as a contaminant. Remember, with disseminated *Candida* you do want to look for endophthalmitis and liver and splenic lesions which she did not have at this time. Note, that sometimes the liver/spleen lesions may not occur until after her neutropenia has resolved!

205. Answer: C

The correct answer is Pyrazinamide (PZA). Note that hyperuricemia is common but gout is rare. PZA along with INH and Rifampin will cause hepatitis also. INH can cause peripheral neuropathy. Rash is seen with PZA and Ethambutol. And with Ethambutol the thing to look out for is optic neuritis particularly manifested by changes in vision especially with colors.

206. Answer: B

The correct answer is *Mycobacterium tuberculosis*. He most likely has AIDS. He has scattered lymphadenopathy with lower lobe infiltrates. He does not have severe hypoxia or disseminated diffuse disease on CXR helping to differentiate from *Pneumocystis*. The hilar adenopathy helps you lean toward tuberculosis also. The other organisms are much less likely. Look for *Bartonella* with skin lesions—patients with HIV get bacillary angiomatosis; *Rhodococcus* is possible but much rarer than *Mycobacterium tuberculosis*. He has no travel history to suggest that Coccidioidomycosis should be considered.

207. Answer: B

The correct answer is oral fluconazole. She has cystitis with yeast likely to be sensitive to fluconazole and more than likely due to the stupid urethral catheter which should have been removed days ago. You would not subject this girl to amphotericin (ampho-terrible) B and oral administration only works for oral and esophageal candidiasis. Re-insertion of the indwelling urethral catheter is not a good idea as you will likely just perpetuate her symptoms with continued colonization of her bladder.

208. Answer: A

The correct answer is to continue INH, repeat serum aminotransferase measurements in one month or sooner if clinically warranted. Remember that these values can go up to 3x normal WITH SYMPTOMS and 5x normal WITHOUT SYMPTOMS!! before you worry about stopping or changing agents. Also the current guidelines published in June 2000 in the MMWR vol .49; no RR-6 state that routine testing is NOT recommended unless patients have a history of liver disease, have HIV infection, are pregnant, are immediately post-partum (within 3 months of delivery), drink alcohol regularly, take other medications that have potential liver toxicity effects, or are at risk for chronic liver disease.

209. Answer: D

The correct answer is Neurocysticercosis. This term is used for human CNS infection with *Taenia solium* cysts. Most literature involves intracerebral cysts which produce seizures and mass effects. Intraventricular cysts as well as subarachnoid cysts can also occur. Drug therapy with albendazole is the treatment of choice. Sometimes corticosteroids are also required if CNS inflammation is severe or causing symptoms. He does not have HIV. So that really throws *Toxoplasma* and *Cryptococcus* out the window. Lymphoma would be really unusual to give you "cystic" lesions. HSV should not do this normally.

Also, with this, think of someone with seizures who has this lesion but they haven't traveled anywhere. The kicker is that they live with a housekeeper or someone who has the infection and is transmitting it fecal/orally in the house. Usually it is a cook or something like that. Lots of literature on this in the early 90's so be aware of the "cook" from Mexico and a kid or the mother starts to have a seizure disorder after a year or two.

210. Answer: E

The correct answer is Mefloquine, starting one week before his travel and continuing for 4 weeks after returning to the U.S. This is a standard question. Mefloquine is the drug of choice. Remember to start it a week before leaving and continuing for 4 weeks after returning from an endemic area. Chloroquine resistance is too high in Africa to consider its use. Doxycycline for that prolonged period of time in a person who will be exposed to sunlight a lot is not practical from a gastrointestinal standpoint or sunburn standpoint. Primaquine is not used for prophylaxis but is used as an adjuvant treatment for *Plasmodium ovale* and *vivax* to get rid of the "liver" forms of this disease.

211. Answer: C

The correct answer is by causing an IgE mediated reaction against proteins in the sting media. Anaphylaxis due to bee stings, foods and heterologous serum (such as tetanus antitoxin) is likely due to an IgE mediated reaction against the offending protein. In contrast (bad pun sorry), radiocontrast media directly activates these cells to release the mediators of anaphylaxis. Anaphylaxis due to penicillin and other antibiotics is due to IgE recognition of protein-hapten conjugants. Finally, dialysis induces anaphylaxis with complement activation.

212. Answer: A

The correct answer is she had IgE recognition of protein-hapten conjugants. Anaphylaxis due to penicillin and other antibiotics is due to IgE recognition of protein-hapten conjugants. Anaphylaxis due to bee stings, foods and heterologous serum (such as tetanus antitoxin) is likely due to an IgE mediated reaction against the offending protein. In contrast (bad pun sorry), radiocontrast media directly activates these cells to release the mediators of anaphylaxis. Finally, dialysis induces anaphylaxis with complement activation.

213. Answer: D

The correct answer is decongestants/nasal irrigation. This patient presents with a 5-day history of rhinorrhea, sore throat and facial pain. She is afebrile with swollen nasal turbinates on exam. Her symptom complex is most consistent with the common cold. The CDC campaign to limit antibiotic use advises to wait 7-10 days before considering treatment with antibiotics for "sinusitis" for facial pain/persistent congestion. The yellow discharge does not increase the likelihood of a bacterial infection. The best treatment would be to begin saline nasal irrigation and topical decongestants for several days WITHOUT antibiotic treatment.

214. Answer: A

The correct "incorrect" response for this question is they are usually immune responses. Anaphylactoid reactions are all of the choices EXCEPT they are usually NOT immune responses. This was a trick..Jerry had anaphylaxis..but I didn't ask about that..I asked about anaphylactoid reactions!! Anaphylactoid reactions are systemic reactions that have the same symptoms as anaphylaxis. They are NOT IgE-dependent and are usually NOT immune. Radiographic contrast agents and non-steroidal anti-inflammatory drugs are examples of these types of reactions.

215. Answer: B

The correct answer is to give epinephrine 1/1000 0.5cc SQ. Expect at least one of these on the "real" test. Remember that IV steroids are not effective acutely. She is NOT hypotensive so she does not need epinephrine IV and then you would use the 1/10,000 formulation of 5cc with fluid expanders and possibly dopamine if needed. Beta-blockade would be a disaster and you would not want to do that! It will blunt the effect of your epinephrine also! If she had bronchospasm you would consider aminophylline. Use of diphenhydramine and cimetidine is also helpful after the epinephrine.

216. Answer: E

The correct answer is immunotherapy—it is not considered to be of value in managing atopic dermatitis. Patients with atopic dermatitis usually do not tolerate immunotherapy as compared to those with respiratory allergy.

217. Answer: B

The correct answer is serum sickness. This is in contrast to all of the other hypersensitivity reactions— serum sickness CAN occur after the initial injection of a foreign serum without any prior sensitization. Today it is most commonly due to penicillin injections, when the benzylpenicilloyl haptenic determinant (try saying that 3 times really fast—better yet try typing it at all) binds by the beta-lactam ring to autologous proteins to become a complete antigen. It can also follow the stings of insects of the order Hymenoptera (bees, wasps, yellow jackets, hornets).

218. Answer: D

The answer is Cardiologist. This child has Kawasaki disease. Although there can be multiple complications, cardiac involvement (especially coronary aneurysms) is the most important. When Kawasaki disease is suspected, a cardiologist should always be involved. Treatment is IV gamma globulin and salicylate therapy started within 10 days of onset to prevent coronary vascular damage.

219. Answer: D

The correct answer is she will need a repeat dose given in 11 months after her IVIG. She has received a large dose of IVIG (2 grams/kg). As such, you have to wait 11 months before she can receive measles vaccination with MMR. She received the IVIG within 2 weeks of her vaccination and there is a good possibility that her immune response will be muted. Checking her measles titer at 2 weeks will be useless—remember she got TONS of IVIG!! You could wait and check her titers at 11 months—but most would recommend just repeating her MMR then.

220. Answer: A

The correct answer is IgA deficiency. IVIG is contraindicated in IgA deficiency. IVIG can contain small amounts of IgA. If a person with IgA deficiency has been sensitized to IgA they could anaphylax if they received IVIG. All of the other conditions listed are appropriate for IVIG administration.

221. Answer: E

The correct answer is cytoplasmic μ chains—the heavy chain of immunoglobulin M. Pre-B cells lack any membrane-bound immunoglobulin.

222. Answer: B

The correct answer is C1 esterase inhibitor. The classical pathway of complement activation is initiated by an antibody-antigen interaction. The first complement component is C1—a complex composed of 3 proteins. C1 binds to immune complexes with activation mediated by C1q. Active C1 then initiates the cleavage and concomitant activation of C4 and C2. A plasma protease inhibitor—known as C1 esterase inhibitor, destroys the activated C1. Patients like Mr. Dude may develop angioedema. It is usually an autosomal disorder but can be acquired in some malignant and autoimmune diseases. Danazol is very helpful in treating this disorder, as it will increase the level of C1 esterase inhibitor.

223. Answer: A

The correct answer is monthly intravenous immunoglobulin. She has common variable immunodeficiency. B-cells can recognize antigen and multiply, but fail to differentiate to the immunoglobulin-secreting stage. Nodular lymphoid hyperplasia and splenomegaly is usually found in these patients. These patients have PAN-hypogammaglobulinemia. Think about this disease in anyone who presents with chronic pulmonary infections, unexplained bronchiectasis (like Margaret), recurrent Giardia, and atrophic gastritis. The therapy for common variable immunodeficiency is replacement of immunoglobulin—mainly immunoglobulin G—with IVIG. You would like the level to reach 500 mg/dl.

224. Answer: D

The correct answer is ataxia-telangiectasia syndrome. This is an autosomal recessive disorder that is associated with abnormal thymic development. The progressive cerebellar ataxia and telangiectasias are obviously hallmarks for this disease. The gene responsible is located on chromosome 11. The defect in the gene results in an inability to repair damaged DNA. I threw in the adenosine deaminase deficiency just to remind you that it is NOT associated with ataxia-telangiectasia syndrome but is associated with severe combined immunodeficiency.

225. Answer: A

The correct answer is systemic mastocytosis. She has a syndrome characterized by mast cell infiltration of the skin (the small bumps that are itchy—known as urticaria pigmentosa), and gastrointestinal mucosa involvement. Usually the spleen and liver are also involved. The ulcer she developed is from histamine-mediated hypersecretion of gastric acid. You can confirm the diagnosis by measuring urine for histamine metabolites or by measuring increased levels of serum histamine or mast cell-derived neutral protease tryptase.

226. Answer: E

The correct answer is Henoch-Schönlein purpura (HSP). He has the classic findings of purpura that is confined to the buttocks and lower extremities. Additionally he has signs of gastrointestinal involvement as well as glomerulonephritis. Most of the time HSP is self-limited but occasionally it can progress to a chronic form.

227. Answer: A

The correct answer is they lack readily detectable immunoglobulin of ANY class on their membranes. Remember that detectable immunoglobulin is found on B-cells.

228. Answer: E

The correct answer is that all of the statements are true. I threw this one in, just so you could remember all of the wonderful things that IgA does for us—and you might get tested on during the ABP torture (er..I mean testing) session. It is really quite under appreciated compared to IgG—the most common immunoglobulin in SERUM and IgM—the principal immunoglobulin in the primary immune response.

229. Answer: C

The correct answer is isolated IgA deficiency. Isolated IgA deficiency is the most common immunodeficiency and has an incidence between 1:600 and 1:800. People with this disorder have a normal or reduced number of B cells with surface IgA, but have an overabundance of immature cells that express both IgA and IgM. The problem is that it appears that the cells cannot secrete IgA effectively. Thus there is a reduced amount of serum as well as secretory IgA. About 30-40% of people with IgA deficiency have antibodies to IgA—thus if they get exposed to IgA (like in blood products or IVIG) they will anaphylax.

230. Answer: B

The correct answer is most immune complexes are removed by the reticuloendothelial system. Deposition of the immune complexes in tissues, other than the reticuloendothelial system, is what results in signs and symptoms of immune-complex disease. It appears that persistence of complexes is required for the development of renal disease. Immune complex mediated vascular damage can lead to cutaneous necrotizing vasculitis.

231. Answer: A

The correct answer is mature red blood cells. All other cells of the body express Class I HLA antigens. Remember that Class I HLA antigens are encoded at the A, B, and C loci of the human major histocompatibility complex on chromosome 6. The Class I HLA antigens are useful in predicting results for organ transplants.

232. Answer: C

The correct answer is that it is associated with a low IgM. Usually these patients have HIGH IgA and IgE. They are at increased risk for infection and they can be treated successfully with bone marrow transplantation.

233. Answer: D

The correct answer is Kawasaki Disease. She has all of the classic findings: She has fever which is a requirement and then she has 1) conjunctivitis; 2) erythematous mouth and pharynx, strawberry tongue, and red, cracked lips; 3) a generalized rash; 4) changes to the peripheral extremities consisting of induration of the hands and feet with red palms and soles; and 5) a unilateral cervical lymph node enlarged to more than 1.5 cm in diameter. Patients have to have fever and at least 4 of 5 findings. If there are less than 4 classic findings then a diagnosis of atypical Kawasaki should be considered. Treatment is with IVIG 2 grams/kg x 1 time dose over 12-14 hours and aspirin in high doses initially followed by low maintenance doses. Usually this occurs in children under the age of 5; however, cases in teenagers have been reported.

234. Answer: D

The correct answer is dermatomyositis. She has the characteristic heliotrope rash and Gottron plaques. The proximal muscle weakness along with the elevated CPK, the muscle biopsy showing necrosis, and the EMG findings are also classically described. Treatment is usually with high dose prednisone and should continue until symptoms improve and serum enzymes are normal. Then patients may remain on maintenance prednisone for several years to reduce risk of exacerbation.

235. Answer: A

The correct answer is nephritis. This is generally one of the determinations of prognosis in children with SLE. The major determinant of mortality in children is the extent of renal involvement and the degree of immunosuppression resulting from therapy. None of the other items listed is particularly a poor sign.

236. Answer: B

The correct answer is if the RF is positive, she will likely have more aggressive disease. There are 2 types of polyarticular JRA. The type is determined based on the RF being positive or negative. A positive RF indicates a more aggressive disease and is associated with HLA DR4 and rheumatoid nodules. Either form will likely have a positive ANA. The RF positive form more commonly occurs at an older age.

237. Answer: C

The correct answer is repeat ANA, anti-dsDNA titers, anti-centromere and anti-SCL70. The patient most likely has primary Raynaud's. Approximately 20% of younger women with primary Raynaud's have a positive ANA and this is not always an appropriate screening test. However, given the fact that her ANA is known to be positive, it would be appropriate and reassuring to exclude a secondary process. Her symptoms do not particularly suggest a connective tissue disease process, but a repeat ANA would be appropriate because of variations from lab to lab. The specific serologies for lupus including anti-dsDNA and SM would be reasonable. So, too, would be an anti-centromere to rule out CREST and an anti-SCL70 to exclude scleroderma. If these last two tests were found to be positive, then a further screening to include manometry, ECHO, etc., would be appropriate. The negative vital capillaroscopy is indeed reassuring. What the heck is <u>that</u> you may ask? It is viewing the cutaneous capillaries at the base of the fingernail through the low power of the microscope. AH..ok. What ever you say.

238. Answer: E

The correct answer is check baseline labs to include CBC, Sed rate, RF and aspirate one of the knees. This patient has a classic reactive arthritis, probably acquired through the gastrointestinal route. She provides no history to suggest any other reactive features to include either urethritis or conjunctivitis. IV antibiotics would obviously have been inappropriate. It would be more appropriate to aspirate the joint and have baseline labs checked before proceeding to systemic corticosteroids or local joint injection.

239. Answer: A

The correct answer is arthralgia. The 5 major criteria are carditis, polyARTHRITIS, chorea, erythema marginatum, and subcutaneous nodules. The minor manifestations are fever, elevated acute phase reactants (WBC, ESR, C-reactive protein), past history of rheumatic fever, prolonged PR or QT interval on ECG, and arthralgia. Remember 2 Major or 1 major and 2 minor manifestations WITH evidence of recent *Streptococcus pyogenes* infection are suggestive of Rheumatic Fever.

240. Answer: C

The correct answer is chorea. The reason for this is that the interval between Group A Streptococcal infection and chorea is much longer than for any of the other major criterion of acute rheumatic fever. It may be months after the initial infection before chorea may occur as opposed to the usual "weeks" with the other manifestations.

241. Answer: B

The answer is Reiter syndrome. Reiter syndrome is a reactive arthritis plus conjunctivitis and urethritis. It can follow GI or GU (most commonly *Chlamydia* or gonorrhea) infections. It is most likely caused by a cross-reactivity of T-lymphocytes to antigens in the joints. There is no specific treatment except to relieve pain. The arthritis can last weeks or become chronic.

242. Answer: D

The answer is lavage the eyes for about 15 minutes, then go directly to the emergency room. Chemical burns to the eye are ocular emergencies. Alkali burns often cause penetrating corneal injuries, while acid burns tend to cause more localized tissue damage. Severe alkali burns often cause corneal opacification. Emergency treatment involves immediate saline or water irrigation of the affected eye for 15-30 minutes. This should be done prior to transporting the child to the emergency room where irrigation should then resume. pH strips should be used to assure maintenance of an ocular pH of 7.3-7.7. Ophthalmologic evaluation should then occur.

243. Answer: C

The answer is rapidly administer 20 ml/kg of isotonic fluids IV. This patient's symptoms of tachycardia, poor perfusion, delayed capillary refill, cool extremities, and hypotension (defined for >1 year as systolic BP < 70 + [2 x age in years]) are consistent with shock. Shock is defined as a condition in which tissue perfusion is inadequate to meet metabolic demands. When signs of poor perfusion are present with a normal blood pressure, the child is in compensated shock. Poor perfusion with hypotension is decompensated shock. This child is in decompensated shock, and the condition is life-threatening. This child needs immediate fluid resuscitation with an isotonic fluid. The child's breathing and heart rate are adequate at this point, so intubation and epinephrine are not needed at this point. Dopamine is sometimes used to help with perfusion, but not as first-line therapy.

244. Answer: A

The answer is make the child "NPO" and refer for inpatient EGD. Ingestion of household cleaning products is a common cause of corrosive esophagitis in young children. Alkali products can cause a severe liquefaction necrosis that involves all layers of the esophagus. Since alkalis may have no taste, children may ingest large volumes. Symptoms of ingestion include salivation, refusal to drink, nausea, vomiting, epigastric pain, oral burns or ulcerations, fever, leukocytosis, and esophageal perforation. Later, esophageal strictures may occur causing dysphagia and weight loss. Emergency treatment involves dilution of the corrosive material with oral administration of large amounts of water or milk. Induced emesis, gastric lavage, and attempted neutralization are contraindicated. Airway edema may necessitate intubation or tracheostomy. No further oral intake should be attempted by the child. EGD should be performed within 48 hours of the injury. In children with significant esophageal injury, long term follow up is recommended to evaluate for the development of esophageal strictures.

245. Answer: B

The answer is plain film x-rays of the orbit. Orbital floor fractures, or blowout fractures occur when an object larger than the orbit strike the orbit. Signs and symptoms of an orbital floor fracture include limitation of upward gaze, lower lid ecchymosis, nosebleed, orbital emphysema, and hypesthesia of the ipsilateral cheek and upper lip. The Waters view plain film radiography is best for demonstrating an orbital floor fracture, although CT can be used. Treatment includes immediate surgical referral if entrapment of the extraocular muscles occurs. Otherwise, the child may be treated with nasal decongestants and ice packs.

246. Answer: E

The answer is naloxone. This patient suffers from opiate intoxication and exhibits the opiate toxidrome of coma, respiratory depression, and miosis. Other symptoms (some of which this patient exhibits) include hypotension, bradycardia or tachycardia, delayed gastric emptying, arrhythmias, pulmonary edema, and circulatory collapse.

Treatment includes respiratory support, ECG monitoring, naloxone administration, and treatment of shock if present.

247. Answer: A

The answer is supportive care. This describes the bite of a brown recluse spider (*Loxosceles species*) which usually goes unnoticed initially. The venom contains proteins that lyse cell walls. Within 2 hours, a painful blue macule with surrounding inflammation appears at the site, followed by systemic symptoms including fever, chills, nausea, and vomiting. Within 1-2 days, a hemorrhagic blister forms which then becomes a necrotic ulcer (usually 1-2 cm in diameter). Most bites resolve with supportive care, but if the patient has severe systemic symptoms, admission to the hospital for observation and pain control is warranted. Local wound care for the ulcerative lesion is usually sufficient.

248. Answer: C

The correct "incorrect" answer is you should get the first plasma level of acetaminophen at 2 hours post-ingestion to determine need for treatment. Signs and symptoms of acetaminophen poisoning include nausea, vomiting, and malaise within the first 24 hours, clinical improvement over the next 48 hours, followed by evidence of hepatic dysfunction. The plasma level should be drawn at 4 hours post-ingestion and plotted on the nomogram. The need for treatment cannot be extrapolated based on a level before 4 hours. Charcoal can be used if started within 1-2 hours of ingestion. At therapeutic doses, a small amount of acetaminophen is metabolized by P-450 enzymes to the highly reactive metabolite NAPQI. It combines with glutathione to form a harmless conjugate. When hepatic stores of glutathione are depleted to less than 70% of normal, NAPQI combines with hepatic molecules causing cellular damage. NAC, which is the antidote, works by restoring hepatic glutathione.

249. Answer: D

The correct answer is organophosphate poisoning. In addition to the above-mentioned symptoms, organophosphate poisoning can also produce dizziness, headache, blurred vision, hyperglycemia, cyanosis, convulsions, and coma in severe cases. These findings are caused by cholinesterase inhibition that results in accumulation of acetylcholine. Symptoms usually occur within 12 hours of exposure. Cholinesterase levels of red cells are measured to determine significant exposure (below 25% normal). Treatment consists of atropine and pralidoxime (cholinesterase reactivator).

250. Answer: D

The correct answer is to administer calcium gluconate – This patient has acute renal failure secondary to rhabdomyolysis, and has developed a bradyarrhythmia secondary to hyperkalemia. The clinical presentation and the markedly elevated CPK are adequate to establish the diagnosis; even before the urine myoglobin is available. It is important to realize that this test may be negative depending on when it is obtained. The presence of 4+ blood without red blood cells on microscopic examination associated with granular casts is characteristic of ATN associated with rhabdomyolysis. In patients who become oliguric, particularly with severe muscle injury, hyperkalemia can be a potentially lethal complication. Initially, T waves may become peaked, but as hyperkalemia worsens, patients may develop variable degrees of heart block, eventually resulting in third degree heart block and severe conduction delays. Such patients are at risk of cardiac arrest. The first step in the emergency treatment of hyperkalemia is to administer calcium to stabilize the cardiac membrane. This can be administered as 10 ml of 10% calcium gluconate over ten minutes, followed by glucose and insulin, which will then push potassium back into the cells until the total potassium burden can be removed through dialysis or other therapy.

It is incorrect to administer Kayexalate enemas – Kayexalate is inappropriate for the emergency therapy of hyperkalemia. The onset of action is several hours and Kayexalate should only be used in life threatening hyperkalemia after treatment with calcium, glucose and insulin or other agents has been administered, particularly if dialysis is not available.

Initiate dialysis therapy is not correct – hyperkalemia and acute renal failure are clearly an indication for dialysis; however, medical therapy should always be the initial therapy while awaiting dialysis, and in patients with EKG changes, calcium should be administered. It would be appropriate to obtain urgent consultation in such a patient but it would be incumbent on the treating physicians to manage the patient medically until dialysis could be initiated.

Temporary pacemaker placement is not indicated – recognition of this patient's heart block as being due to hyperkalemia is essential in the appropriate management. In the setting of rhabdomyolysis and acute renal failure, the diagnosis of hyperkalemia as the cause of heart block must be considered and therefore the heart block will resolve once hyperkalemia is appropriately treated. Even in patients who demonstrate hemodynamic instability, immediate treatment of hyperkalemia typically resolves heart block and therefore pacing is usually not necessary.

To perform fasciotomies is incorrect. – while fasciotomy may be necessary in patients with compartment syndromes and persistent rhabdomyolysis, this would not be appropriate initial therapy with life threatening arrhythmia secondary to hyperkalemia.

251. Answer: A

The correct answer is chemical pneumonitis. CNS changes can be seen but are less common than pneumonitis and generally require higher doses. Liver disease is usually not a problem. Aplastic anemia is not a problem.

252. Answer: C

The correct answer is to transfuse 2 units packed red blood cells. This patient is still only partially resuscitated with evidence for both hemorrhagic shock and the hyperdynamic phase of SIRS (systemic inflammatory response syndrome). Most important is the continued acidosis which is predominantly a metabolic acidosis and presumably a lactic acidosis indicating inadequate tissue perfusion. The best way to continue the resuscitation is to improve oxygen delivery (DO2) to the tissues and monitor the ABG and lactate level to assess improvement. Oxygen delivery is determined by cardiac output, hemoglobin and oxygen <u>saturation</u>. In this case, the CO is already high and the oxygen saturation with a PO2 of 85 is at least 90%. Increasing the PO2 will not provide much more hemoglobin saturation. Therefore, the best way to improve oxygen delivery is to increase the hemoglobin through additional packed red cell transfusions. Increasing the minute ventilation to compensate for the metabolic acidosis will only mask the problem. Dobutamine will reduce the systemic vascular resistance even more resulting in further hypotension. Dopamine will increase the blood pressure and cause further tachycardia with no improvement in oxygen delivery to the tissues.

253. Answer: A

The correct answer is High Cardiac output, Low Systemic Vascular resistance and Low Wedge pressure. Utilizing a Swan Ganz catheter to generate a hemodynamic profile of shock, such as above, is a reasonable question for the exam. They may even throw in more data such as Pulmonary Artery pressure, mixed venous oxygen saturation and even Left Ventricular Stroke Volume to foul you up. Stick to the parameters above and you should be able to narrow down the answer sufficiently.

Remember the hallmark of early, "warm" sepsis is a hyperdynamic heart (increased cardiac output) coupled with a <u>very low systemic vascular resistance</u>. Typically the patient in early septic shock is volume depleted and "third spacing" a considerable amount of the fluids given for resuscitation due to the low systemic vascular resistance. In all the other entities above, the systemic vascular resistance is high as it is the only thing holding the blood pressure together!

Hypovolemic shock, whether hemorrhagic or intravascular volume depletion is characterized by a low wedge pressure, a reduced cardiac output and a high SVR.
Cardiogenic shock is defined by a low cardiac output, high filling pressures (think CHF) and a high SVR. Obstructive shock is typified by a massive PE or a tension pneumothorax. There is reduced cardiac filling, reduced cardiac output and a high SVR. In pericardial tamponade the filling pressures will be normal as a reduced volume is acted on by a decreased compliance of the ventricular wall.

254. Answer: D

The correct answer is Methylene blue. This patient presents with hypotension, and cyanosis. He was at a party when the symptoms started. This presentation is suggestive of nitrite abuse. He most likely used amyl nitrite ("poppers") at the party. The nitrite induces methemoglobinemia which causes the cyanosis unresponsive to oxygen administration. Administration of methylene blue will reduce ferric iron to its ferrous state, resolving the methemoglobinemia.

255. Answer: A

The correct answer is imaging of the brain and ophthalmologic evaluation. A port wine stain on the face may be an indication of Sturge-Weber disease which occurs sporadically with a frequency of 1 in 50,000 births. Sturge-Weber disease may be associated with facial nevus, intracranial calcifications, seizures, hemiparesis, ipsilateral glaucoma, and mental retardation. The facial nevus is often unilateral and involves the upper face and eyelid. It may extend over the lower face and trunk, mouth and pharynx. Infants suspected of having Sturge-Weber warrant an ophthalmologic evaluation for glaucoma and neuro imaging to evaluate for intracranial calcifications and structural abnormalities. Approximately 50% of children with Sturge-Weber disease develop mental retardation or learning disabilities. While laser surgery may improve the appearance of the nevus, there is no indication to perform it urgently.

256. Answer: E

The correct answer is you reassure her that this is a self-limited process and that sunlight may help to accelerate remission. This patient has pityriasis rosea, which is a self-limited inflammatory dermatosis of unknown etiology. It is usually characterized by the appearance of a solitary oval patch on the trunk (herald patch), and within 7-14 days, numerous small, oval, pink plaques develop on the trunk, extremities, and neck. These are usually asymptomatic and last for 6 to 8 weeks. The lesions usually follow the lines of skin cleavage (called Christmas tree pattern). No specific treatment is recommended, and complete remission will occur. If present, severe pruritus can be treated with a mid-potency topical corticosteroid. Ultraviolet B irradiation can speed up remission.

257. Answer: C

The correct answer is Erythema toxicum neonatorum (ETN). ETN is the most common pustular rash occurring in up to 70% of full-term infants. Usually lesions appear on the 2nd or 3rd day of life but can appear in up to 2-3 weeks of age. It usually begins with 2-3 mm erythematous blotchy macules and papules, some evolving into yellow pustules on an erythematous base. Lesions may occur on the face, trunk, and proximal extremities and usually fade over 5-7 days. A Wright stain shows eosinophils and occasional neutrophils.

258. Answer: A

The correct answer is topical tretinoin. The diagnosis of acne is established when three of the six lesions of acne are present. The lesions of acne are papules, pustules, open and closed comedones, ice pick scars, hyperpigmented macules, and cystic lesions. If, as in this patient, the majority of the lesions are non-inflammatory, topical retinoids are the treatment of choice because of their keratolytic effect. The other choices listed are not keratolytic, and thus would be less effective for the patient described. And you wouldn't want to use topical interferon for acne!

259. Answer: D

The correct answer is topical steroids do produce multiple side effects. Topical steroids had been the mainstay of therapy of treatment for atopic skin prior to the development of immune modulators such as pimecrolimus and tacrolimus. Although both of the new drugs have local side effects such as burning and stinging, topical steroids can cause striae, atrophy, telangiectasia, pigmentary changes and acneform skin eruptions. Lubrication alone would not be expected to produce local side effects.

260. Answer: D

The correct answer is erythema nodosum. In addition to sarcoidosis, erythema nodosum can be associated with streptococcal infections, inflammatory bowel disease, tuberculosis, and drug allergy. The association of erythema nodosum, arthritis, anterior uveitis, and hilar adenopathy due to sarcoidosis is termed Lofgren's Syndrome, and is usually associated with good prognosis. Although the classical Lofgren's syndrome is a tetrad, the term is commonly applied when a patient presents with only sarcoidosis and erythema nodosum. The lack of appropriate history, and the appearance of the biopsy exclude the other diagnoses. Erythema nodosum can be treated with non-steroidal anti-inflammatory drugs, topical or systemic steroids, or immunosuppressive agents.

261. Answer: A

The correct answer is Impetigo vulgaris. The trauma caused by scratching had broken the skin and permitted bacterial invasion and secondary infection. Most community acquired skin infections are due to *Streptococcal* or *Staphylococcal species*. Impetigo vulgaris is most often caused by *Staphylococci*. Erythema nodosum most often presents as tender nodules on the pre-tibial surfaces of the legs. The diagnosis of acne vulgaris requires the presence of at least three of the six characteristic lesions. In general, drug eruptions most commonly start on the chest, abdomen or the back.

262. Answer: D

The correct answer is Hepatitis C. Hepatitis C is frequently found in association with PCT. In addition to vesicles of the skin, there can also be increased pigmentation, increased fragility, and milia formation. Patients with PCT also have an increased incidence of liver cirrhosis and liver cancer. Acanthosis nigricans and paraneoplastic pemphigus are not associated with PCT.

263. Answer: C

The correct answer is Herpetic infections. Exfoliative dermatitis is not associated with herpes simplex or *herpes zoster*. It is frequently seen as an allergic reaction to such drugs as sulfonamides, anti-malarials, penicillin, phenytoin, and barbiturates. It has also been associated with benign skin diseases such as atopic dermatitis, or malignant processes such as mycosis fungoides. Exfoliative dermatitis has also been found in association with solid tumors. No matter what the etiology, the skin biopsy is often non-specific. The course and prognosis of exfoliative dermatitis is related to the course of the underlying process.

264. Answer: B

The correct answer is to refer her for excisional biopsy of the lesion. Superficial spreading melanoma is the most common type of melanoma, and comprises seventy percent of all melanomas. It is found predominantly in young people who burn rather than tan. The favored location is the back of the legs on women and the backs of men. When such a lesion is identified, referral is indicated for simple excision and histological evaluation. Based on the depth of invasion, re-excision margins are decided and the patient's prognosis is determined. A punch biopsy of the brown area will show melanocytes in the epidermis, which may or may not be malignant and could result in an inaccurate diagnosis. Likewise, liquid nitrogen will only remove the superficial portion of the tumor, leaving the dermal portion to proliferate and metastasize. Whenever a melanoma is suspected, intervention is indicated because malignant melanoma is a life threatening disease. By the year 2010 it is estimated that one in fifty people will have melanoma.

265. Answer: E

The correct answer is sparfloxacin. This patient developed a rash after taking an antibiotic while on vacation in Hawaii. The distribution of the rash is strongly suggestive of a photosensitivity reaction. The quinolones have a varying phototoxicity profile, with sparfloxacin the most phototoxic. Norfloxacin is minimally phototoxic. Amoxicillin/clavulanate and nitrofurantoin do not cause phototoxic reactions.

266. Answer: A

The correct answer is cutaneous candidal infection. Typically these infections occur at sites that are chronically wet and macerated such as an intertriginous area that requires frequent water exposure (like Ms. Times). Treatment would involve a topical agent such as topical clotrimazole.

267. Answer: A

The correct answer is dyshidrotic eczema. Hand dermatitis is quite common in individuals who wash their hands frequently and Lynn has a common variant of this. The finding of highly pruritic vesicles on the sides of the fingers is helpful in making this diagnosis. *Lichen planus* is a disorder with papulosquamous pruritic lesions that have a purplish hue. Zoster would present as a group of vesicles on an erythematous base. Atopic dermatitis would be more likely if she had a history of asthma or disease during childhood.

268. Answer: C

The correct answer is Osler-Rendu-Weber disease. All of this stuff is identifiable by the type of telangiectasia!! Know this: Linear telangiectasia on the face—actinically damaged skin; Broad telangiectasia—scleroderma associated with the CREST variant; Periungual telangiectasia—SLE, scleroderma, dermatomyositis; spider-like telangiectasia—Osler-Rendu-Weber disease.

269. Answer: C

The correct answer is syphilis. He has a classic rash of secondary syphilis. The palms and sole involvement is the classic "hallmark" for this disease. Chancre is commonly on the penis but depending upon sexual practices it can be the pharynx or anus.

270. Answer: A

The correct "incorrect" answer is folate deficiency. He has vitiligo, which are macules that are completely lacking in pigment. It is generally a hereditary condition. Most cases are not associated with other disease processes; however those listed besides folate deficiency have been described with this condition.

271. Answer: D

The answer is give IVF with 20-40 mEq/L KCL to correct electrolyte/acid-base imbalance. This baby has projectile non-bilious vomiting that has gotten progressively worse with no other symptoms. This should make you think of pyloric stenosis, especially in a Caucasian first-born male. An ultrasound would be the test to confirm the diagnosis. Lab findings would show a hypochloremic metabolic alkalosis. After diagnosis, you would need to consult a surgeon, but pyloromyotomy cannot be performed until the dehydration and electrolyte/acid-base disturbance is corrected. This usually takes 24-48 hours. Since there is potassium depletion with hypochloremic metabolic alkalosis, KCL should be added to IVF.

272. Answer: A

The answer is Crohn disease. It is a chronic inflammatory bowel disease that involves any portion of the GI tract from mouth to anus. There are many presentations of Crohn disease depending on location of involvement. Children usually present with ileum and colon involvement. Those with ileocolitis will usually present with crampy abdominal pain and diarrhea, sometimes with blood. Ileitis may present with right lower quadrant pain alone. Colitis may present with bloody diarrhea, tenesmus, and urgency. Although diarrhea is a common symptom, patients can present in other ways such as this patient who mainly had large bulky stools instead of diarrhea.

Ileal involvement, strictures, fistulas, skip lesions, and transmural involvement are all common features. Systemic symptoms are more common in Crohn disease than in ulcerative colitis. Fever, malaise, and easy fatigability are common. Growth failure may occur. Perianal disease (including abscess, fistula, and tags) is common. Extraintestinal symptoms can include oral aphthous ulcers, arthritis, erythema nodosum, gallstones, and kidney stones. Rectal disease rarely occurs.

Diagnosis is made by either colonoscopy or radiologic studies depending on anticipated area of disease. Colonoscopy with biopsy is more helpful in evaluating colon disease.
Treatment consists of (1) anti-inflammatory agents—steroids for small bowel involvement and aminosalicylates for colon disease, (2) immunomodulators, and (3) nutritional therapy including total parenteral nutrition if needed. Surgical treatment should be reserved for localized disease that is unresponsive to medical treatment. Reoperation is very likely. This is a chronic disease and symptoms recur despite adequate treatment.

273. Answer: A

The correct answer is *Campylobacter jejuni*. The organism described in the stool culture is *Campylobacter*. It is treated with erythromycin. Puppies and kittens are common sources. So are chickens, turkey and other fowl. By many reports this is the most common cause of enteric diarrhea in the U.S.!!

274. Answer: D

The correct answer is antigliadin antibodies and IgA-endomysial antibodies. Celiac disease should come to mind when the symptoms present after the introduction of cereal and solids (usually between 6-24 months of age). This disorder causes small bowel mucosal damage resulting from gluten sensitivity. Gluten is found in wheat, rye, and barley. Most patients present with diarrhea. Some may just have failure to thrive and vomiting. Irritability and anorexia are common. Patients can have abdominal distention and muscle wasting. Anemia and hypoproteinemia are common. Antigliadin antibodies and particularly IgA-endomysial antibodies are useful screening tests. Small bowel biopsy showing short, flat villi, deepened crypts, and lymphocytes in the epithelial layer (seen by light microscopy) confirm the diagnosis. Treatment consists of a gluten-free diet for life.

275. Answer: A

The correct answer is Pill-induced esophagitis. In adolescents, pill-induced esophagitis is common especially if they do not take the time to use water to swallow pills. Doxycycline is one of the classic drugs to do this. Other common drugs associated with this include aspirin, nonsteroidals such as ibuprofen, iron pills, potassium supplements and alendronate (for post-menopausal osteoporosis). Scleroderma is very unlikely in a 16-year-old male without other symptoms. Gastroesophageal reflux would not generally cause this type of isolated symptom. Cocaine abuse is not associated with isolated dysphagia. Bulimia could be associated with dysphagia but he has no other signs or symptoms of this illness.

276. Answer: C

The correct answer is Serum Gastrin level. Several issues should make you think about Zollinger-Ellison syndrome (ZES). Note, his ulcer is in an unusual location; generally any ulcer past the duodenal bulb should make you think about ZES. Also, he has severe esophagitis, which can be seen in regular ulcers but with the finding of the EGD makes ZES more likely. Additionally, his family history is quite strong and he has been having diarrhea - another hallmark of this syndrome. Although diarrhea often occurs concomitantly with acid peptic disease, it may also occur **independent** of an ulcer. Etiology of the diarrhea is multifactorial, resulting from marked volume overload to the small bowel, pancreatic enzyme inactivation by acid, and damage of the intestinal epithelial surface by acid. Occasionally you can have mild malabsorption of nutrients and vitamins. The diarrhea may also have a secretory component due to the direct stimulatory effect of gastrin on enterocytes or the co-secretion of additional hormones from the tumor, such as vasoactive intestinal peptide.

Gastric acid hypersecretion is responsible for the signs and symptoms observed in patients with ZES. Peptic ulcer is the most common clinical manifestation, occurring in over 90% of gastrinoma patients. Other clinical situations that should create suspicion of gastrinoma are ulcers refractory to standard medical therapy, ulcer recurrence after acid-reducing surgery, or ulcers presenting with frank complications (bleeding, obstruction, and perforation).

277. Answer: E

The correct answer is air contrast barium enema and enteroclysis. She has symptoms consistent with Crohn's disease. A barium enema and enteroclysis will confirm disease location and show evidence of intestinal complications. Lower endoscopy (with or without upper endoscopy) could also be done to confirm the diagnosis. Early in the disease process the barium enema shows thickened folds and aphthous ulcerations. Later, "cobblestoning" from longitudinal and transverse ulcerations most frequently involves the small bowel. As the disease progresses, strictures and fistulas are seen. Skip lesions are seen in Crohn's disease. With her prolonged history and initial negative stool testing, it is not necessary to repeat ova and parasite testing again. An MRI would be helpful if you were concerned about an abscess but currently her symptoms are fairly mild and no evidence exists for this. Endoscopic laparotomy is invasive and not indicated at this stage of diagnosis. A rectal biopsy is contraindicated and will not provide any helpful information for Crohn's disease.

278. Answer: E

The correct answer is stop sulfasalazine and use another agent for control of his disease. Sulfasalazine is split into sulfapyridine and mesalamine. The problem is the sulfapyridine can cause reversible infertility in men. The best answer is to stop the sulfasalazine and prescribe another agent or attempt a trial of therapy since he has not had a problem in over 5 years. Once he has achieved "success" then you could restart the sulfasalazine. Formal urologic evaluation is not indicated at this point. Also we have found that his sperm count is abnormally low and this explains why they are not conceiving. His wife does not need to undergo any testing. Also, since we have a reversible cause for his infertility and he is "functioning" properly it is unnecessary to proceed with further workup. It wouldn't hurt to try boxers instead of briefs but it is unlikely to make a difference in this case..unless his wife finds them attractive while his sperm count returns to normal.

279. Answer: E

The correct answer is recommend referral to surgery. Even though he has been doing well until recently, the finding of high-grade dysplasia in flat mucosa indicates that colon cancer is possibly imminent and removal of his complete colon will be curative. It is difficult to think about this in someone who has had relatively mild ulcerative colitis. Additionally, if you had found a mass lesion that showed dysplasia, that would indicate that complete colectomy was indicated. Once you are at this stage, repeat colonoscopy is not helpful and will just prolong the inevitable.

280. Answer: A

The answer is no antibiotic therapy. With uncomplicated *Salmonella*, gastroenteritis antibiotic therapy is not indicated. If you treat her with antibiotics you risk prolonging her shedding as well as increasing risk of resistance. Remember, *Shigella* you treat; *Salmonella* you generally don't. Exceptions are the very old, the very young, and the immunocompromised. We treat them with antibiotics because the risk that the *Salmonella* may disseminate or cause more extensive problems is greater than the risk of prolonged shedding.

281. Answer: E

The Answer is none of the choices are correct. Recent information has shown that starting antibiotics in patients with *E. coli* 0157:H7 actually INCREASES the risk of HUS (Hemolytic uremic syndrome). Therefore, supportive care is all that is indicated for this patient. Antibiotics are absolutely contraindicated!!

282. Answer: A

The answer is *Campylobacter jejuni*. This patient has classic Guillain-Barré syndrome. Classically this has been described as a syndrome that is spontaneous. However, *Campylobacter* enteritis is linked to about 1/3 of cases. The other organisms listed are not associated with this syndrome. Of note, as in this case, humans can get *Campylobacter* from their pets, especially dogs; conversely dogs have become infected from their owners.

283. Answer: B

The correct answer is phenolphthalein abuse. Note that she has a normal physical examination. The only positive laboratory value is that little sodium hydroxide test which indicates that she is abusing phenolphthalein. You can confirm this with specific urine tests also for this agent. The bisacodyl could be confirmed also by urine testing. IBS is a diagnosis of exclusion and we have found another etiology for her symptoms. Carcinoid is a rare cause of diarrhea; she does not have any of the other symptoms such as flushing, tachycardia, and explosive diarrhea. Colonoscopy and EGD are reserved for the final stage of workup of chronic diarrhea and are not indicated at this point, particularly in light of our findings of phenolphthalein abuse.

284. Answer: A

The correct answer is iron deficiency anemia. Remember that iron is almost completely absorbed in the duodenum. With celiac sprue this is one of the main sites of malabsorption. B-12 deficiency is very common with tropical sprue but not celiac sprue. Folate deficiency is also less likely to be a problem. Celiac sprue exacerbation would not be responsible for anemia of this degree with heme negative stools and no history of blood in the stool. Primary intestinal lymphoma is a rare late complication of celiac sprue—and the key words here are RARE and LATE—so not a concern for this 18-year-old leprechaun at this point.

285. Answer: D

The answer is abdominal CT scan. She has a known history of diverticulitis (that is what that crazy picture is from last year) and now with the findings of rebound tenderness and involuntary abdominal rigidity, this indicates the possibility of an abscess or perforation of a diverticulum. Emergent CT scan (or ultrasound) should be done to evaluate for this possibility. Colonoscopy and barium enema should be avoided during the active stage. If an abscess is found, then drainage is necessary either with radiologic guidance or surgical intervention. Bowel rest is indicated, but you must rule out the possibility of something more severe such as abscess or perforation. A bleeding scan is not indicated, as she has no evidence of a severe bleed.

286. Answer: A

The correct answer is reflux esophagitis. Odynophagia usually relates to acute esophageal injury from medications (e.g. Doxycycline) or infections like Herpes or Candida. Very rarely would reflux esophagitis lead to odynophagia. The appearance above is most consistent with a herpetic infection. Most cases of Herpes esophagitis in the otherwise competent host are due to reactivation of a late Herpes infection rather than primary infection. These are often brought out by high doses of corticosteroids. Biopsies from the edge of the ulcer are helpful, and the tissue should be sent for culture and histology. These patients may respond even without antiviral therapy, especially if the steroids can be discontinued.

287. Answer: D

The correct answer is check the stool for *Clostridium difficile* toxin before initiating therapy. This is a case of ulcerative colitis that has developed a secondary *Clostridium difficile* infection. Many flares of disease activity in patients with IBD may be due to *Clostridium difficile*, and this needs to be aggressively considered. In the appropriate setting, the presence of fecal leukocytes would be good evidence of *C. difficile* infection, for instance, in the hospitalized patient who develops diarrhea after antibiotics. However, in the patient with IBD, who may have fecal leukocytes just related to their disease process, this would not be a reliable sign. Many patients, like this one here, will have a leukocytosis associated with *C. difficile*, although this is not specific. Flexible sigmoidoscopy may reveal pseudomembranes, but is not always diagnostic. Some patients do not have the characteristic pseudomembranous colitis and in some patients, it may be located beyond the range of the flexible sigmoidoscope. In the patient with suspected *C. difficile* colitis, the stool should be sent (preferably 3 specimens) for *C. difficile* toxin. One does not need to send this stool for culture of *C. difficile*. The appropriate therapy is oral Metronidazole.

288. Answer: D

The correct answer is this is likely a *Staphylococcus aureus* food poisoning. These patients have the typical description of *Staph aureus* food poisoning. Patients usually present 4-6 hours after ingestion of the food with nausea, vomiting and diarrhea. These symptoms do not last long, rarely more than 12 hours, but it is not uncommon to have severe dehydration. The *Staph aureus* could have been obtained in the ham or even the deviled eggs. Although undercooked poultry can be a source of *Salmonella*, the incubation period is much longer than what is seen here. Likewise, in *E. coli* 0157, the incubation period is longer, as well. Giardiasis can occur after ingesting Rocky Mountain water, but the symptoms are too severe in this case. And although Marla's deviled eggs would never cause this, someone else's food at the picnic easily could.

The treatment of *Staph aureus* food poisoning revolves around supportive intravenous fluid. This is an ingested toxin, rather than any active bacteria, so there is no value in giving antibiotics.

289. Answer: A

The correct answer is pain farther from the umbilicus is more likely organic. All of the other items listed are false. Most functional abdominal pain in the school age child is periumbilical and poorly localized. Functional pain tends to be more crampy in nature an intermittent crampiness is common. Children who wake at night with abdominal pain are often thought to have organic disease—but it is not uncommon for functional abdominal pain to cause children to wake and seek attention. Pain relieved by meals is more commonly associated with peptic ulcer disease. Pain that occurs shortly after eating is more typically functional but can be associated with biliary or pancreatic disorders. Functional abdominal pain does not usually have associated diarrhea. Vomiting and headaches occur with functional abdominal pain.

290. Answer: E

The correct answer is peritoneal inflammation. This child has intussusception. He needs a radiographic contrast enema for therapeutic reduction. The only contraindications to doing this are signs of peritoneal inflammation (potential necrotic bowel wall) or radiographic appearance of long-standing small intestinal obstruction.

291. Answer: B

The correct "incorrect" answer is it is usually within 2cm of the ileocecal valve. Usually it is within 100cm of the ileocecal valve. All of the other items listed are true.

292. Answer: B

The correct answer is on barium enema, the aganglionic segment is the distal narrowed segment and the normal ganglionic segment is dilated proximally. My goodness, I know that was confusing..but KNOW IT!! The normal part is Proximal! The abnormal part is Distal! The Abnormal part is narrowed! The normal part is Dilated! Put it all together and you get Abnormal: Distal narrowing; Normal: Proximal dilatation. Just remember that "distal and dilated" can't go together—or Double D is not possible.

293. Answer: D

The correct answer is he has acute hepatitis B and past infection with A. He has acute hepatitis B (he is in the "window" period). He only has IgM antibody to Hepatitis B core. He has lost his Hepatitis B surface antigen and will soon develop IgG antibody to Hepatitis B core. He also has IgG to Hepatitis A which means that he has had an old infection that he recovered from. There is no such thing as "chronic Hepatitis A".

On most "screens" for hepatitis, labs do the following tests:
Anti-HAV IgM—looks for acute hepatitis A
HBsAg—looks for acute infection as well as chronic carrier states
Anti-HBc IgM—looks for acute infection in the "window"
Anti-HBc IgG—tells you if a person has been infected with Hepatitis B in the past; does not tell you if they are still infectious-this requires the HBsAg test
Hepatitis C antibody: This just tells you if someone has been infected with hepatitis C; it doesn't tell you status of infection (ie. chronic infected or resolved)

Let's go through the rest of the choices just for fun and how a "screen" would pick this up (come on now..you know you hate this but it will be on the Boards.)

1) Acute hepatitis A and past infection with hepatitis B: Anti-HAV IgM positive; all of the hepatitis B stuff is negative except Hepatitis B Core IgG Antibody
2) Chronic A and Acute B: impossible; remember chronic A does not exist
3) Chronic A and Chronic B: again..impossible for a plain yellow pumpkin..oops that is from Cinderella isn't it? wrong talk about yellow I guess.
4) Neither hepatitis A nor hepatitis B: that would mean that all the studies were negative.

294. Answer: A

The correct answer is by attaching a polyethylene glycol moiety to interferon alpha, there is an increased response rate. Interferon alpha has been the standard therapy for chronic hepatitis C, but treatment has been hampered by its short half-life and wide fluctuations in plasma concentration. A combination of interferon with Ribavirin has been shown to have improved results. Likewise, a recent study demonstrating that PEG interferon Alpha 2a (which is the attachment of a polyethylene glycol moiety to the interferon molecule) causes improved results. When compared to standard interferon, the pegylated interferon had a virologic response at 48 weeks on 69% compared to 28% with interferon alone. Likewise, there was also improvement in the sustained normalization of ALT even at 72 weeks (45% vs 25%). Neutropenia and thrombocytopenia can occasionally complicate the treatment of hepatitis with interferon, but it would be uncommon that this would require cessation of therapy. The most common serious adverse effects are the psychiatric effects including severe depression. Factors which would predict a good response to interferon therapy include lower levels of HCV RNA and an HCV genotype other than Type I.

295. Answer: B

The correct answer is transferrin saturation greater than 50% should prompt further evaluation including HFE gene determination. Hereditary hemochromatosis is a common inherited disorder with a prevalence of 1 in 200 to 1 in 400 in populations of northern European descent. It has an autosomal recessive pattern of inheritance and the gene for the disease, known as the HFE, has recently been discovered. The patients may present with fatigue, malaise, abdominal pain, arthralgias and impotence. However, if discovered by screening of family members or screening of asymptomatic individuals, the majority have no complications such as cirrhosis. Physical examination of patients with hemochromatosis may reveal hepatomegaly and skin hyperpigmentation. Serum iron is generally elevated and the iron saturation is greater than 50%. Values such as these should prompt further gene testing. The serum ferritin is usually abnormal, but can be abnormal in other diseases, such as alcoholic liver disease and HCV. If this patient is found to have hereditary hemochromatosis by genetic testing, then he should undergo weekly therapeutic phlebotomy of 500ml of whole blood until his transferrin saturation is less than 50% and the serum ferritin is less than 50.

296. Answer: E

The correct answer is drug hepatotoxicity. If one includes acetaminophen, then drug hepatotoxicity is clearly the most common cause of acute liver failure in the United States. Acetaminophen is the single most important agent to cause this, although many other drugs may cause this as well. In cases of acetaminophen hepatotoxicity, many of these are due to suicide attempts. However, there are many others who have this due to accidental toxicity due to attempts at pain relief. This can occur if the person over several days is ingesting more than 3gm per day of acetaminophen. Alcoholics seem to be at risk for toxicity even at lower than usual levels of acetaminophen ingestion. Suicide patients often present promptly, but the accidental toxicity patient may have a delayed presentation, and therefore often has a higher mortality. If the patient does present early on, then N-acetyl-cystine may be helpful if administered promptly. Some cases do progress to absolute liver failure which would require transplantation.

297. Answer: A

The correct answer is CXR. Ok, I tried to trick you by putting this in the "GI/Liver section". This guy has pneumonia! Don't ever forget to get a CXR in someone with abdominal pain---it is a favorite trick question on the Boards. Did I trick ya?

298. Answer: C

The correct answer is serum bilirubin reaches maximum values near 6 mg/dl between the 2nd and 4th day in full term infants. Physiologic jaundice does NOT cause damage in healthy full-term infants. The excess bilirubin is due to the infant overproducing bilirubin, combined with immature conjugation and possibly active intestinal reabsorption of bilirubin. Pigment concentrations gradually decline to normal by 2 weeks of age in full term infants.

299. Answer: D

The correct answer is the serum bilirubin reaches maximum concentrations of 15 to 25 mg/dl during the 2nd or 3rd week. Jaundice can persist up to 2 to 3 months! Kernicterus has not been reported in breast-milk jaundice, presumably because peak concentrations of unconjugated bilirubin are reached after the initial week of life in generally healthy infants. Infants with bread-milk jaundice are usually quite active and alert and a finding contrary to this should lead to a workup for other etiologies. The jaundice is due to unconjugated bilirubin only.

300. Answer: E

The correct answer is all of the items listed are true. This is due to an absolute (Type I) or relative (Type II) inherited deficiency of bilirubin UDP-glucuronyl transferase. Type I presents within the first 24 hours of life with rapidly progressive unconjugated bilirubinemia without hemolysis. Bilirubin is unable to be conjugated. Type I's must be administered phototherapy throughout life. Kernicterus can occur at any age! A simple infection such as the common cold, could tip the patient over into kernicterus! Thus, liver transplant is recommended early on for these patients.

Type II can present early or may be delayed for years. The bilirubin can range from normal to 30 mg/dl. Bilirubin UDP-glucuronyl transferase activity may reach 50% of normal. Phenobarbital will reduce the serum bilirubin in Type II patients.

301. Answer: A

The correct answer is exchange blood transfusion and phototherapy are recommended treatments. Poor feeding and absent Moro reflex would make you look for pathologic unconjugated hyperbilirubinemia—BUT not in a non-jaundiced infant! Phototherapy is usually continued until the bilirubin is consistently below 10 mg/dl. Eye shielding is always recommended for any prolonged exposure to sunlight—no matter if you are treating hyperbilirubinemia or going for a nice walk in the park!

302. Answer: A

The correct answer is prothrombin time. Remember I asked for "function" of the liver; not for structural integrity. The transaminases (AST, ALT, which are transaminases) are useful for assessing the structural integrity of the liver—has something caused damage—a virus or a drug. PT and albumin are much better at telling you how the liver is "functioning". PT elevation suggests liver malfunction and albumin abnormalities reflect hepatic capacity for protein synthesis.

303. Answer: E

The correct answer is percutaneous liver biopsy. Note that the bile staining of the stools indicates an intrahepatic process! If there was no bile-staining then it could be intra- or extra-hepatic and you would proceed first to an ultrasound—looking for a choledochus cyst—If it was not present, then you would do hepatic scintigraphy—if this was positive then you would proceed to liver biopsy also.

304. Answer: D

The correct answer is cytomegalovirus. Note, that it is really unusual to find the cytoplasmic inclusions (<5%) but if you do then you have nailed the diagnosis. Generally you have to do urine cultures for CMV and look for specific antibody titer rises. A DNA probe is also commonly available. Hepatitis B and Toxoplasmosis would not give you these inclusions. Aagenes' syndrome is a VERY rare autosomal recessive disorder—it is associated with Norwegian consanguinity—sorry if the "Ingrid" name threw you—although if you knew of this silly syndrome then the rest of the people reading this are glad you missed it—cause that is ridiculous that you knew that syndrome! Byler's disease is another autosomal recessive disorder detected in the Amish—so again pretty rare; even for Board exams in General Pediatrics (hopefully!)!

305. Answer: B

The correct answer is Watson-Alagille syndrome. It is pretty rare only occurring in 2/100,000 live births. About ½ of the kids with paucity of the intrahepatic bile ducts will have the full syndrome; the other ½ will just have neonatal hepatitis or idiopathic infantile cholestasis and are never "diagnosed"; those without the full syndrome usually have a worse prognosis! Treatment is with a low-fat, high protein diet. Pruritus and jaundice can be improved with cholestyramine, phenobarbital, or both. Steatorrhea and bleeding tendencies tend to occur commonly because of poor absorption of fats and vitamin K.

Caroli's disease is cystic dilatation of the intrahepatic bile ducts. It is autosomal recessive. The clinical features are recurrent bouts of cholangitis and abscesses due to bile stasis and gallstone formation within the cysts.

Wolman's disease is a severe disease where the infants are normal at birth but in the first few weeks of life develop severe vomiting and abdominal distention. They have diarrhea, poor weight gain, jaundice and fever. Hepatosplenomegaly is SEVERE within a few days of birth. They have a papulovesicular rash on the face, chest, and neck. They usually die by 3 to 6 months of age.

Gaucher's disease is a group of autosomal recessive sphingolipidoses in which glucocerebroside is stored as a result of deficiency of the enzyme glucocerebroside B-glucosidase. The diagnosis of Gaucher's (Type I) is on the basis of hepatosplenomegaly, increased serum acid phosphatase, and Gaucher cells in the bone marrow.

Ferguson's disease—I just made up in honor of one of MedStudy's outstanding employees.

306. Answer: A

The correct answer is hepatitis B virus is serving as a helper for a viral superinfection. In this case it is likely he has developed a superinfection with hepatitis D. Hepatitis D requires the hepatitis B genome to replicate. Hepatitis C and A cannot facilitate hepatitis D infection. Interferon alpha will not be curative for the superinfection but may help alleviate some of the symptoms.

307. Answer: B

The correct answer is Leukemia. With ITP the platelet count is low, but usually the other CBC indices are normal. Bactrim can cause bone marrow suppression, but does not explain the x-ray findings. A septic picture could present with these lab findings, but this child does not appear ill at all. Lupus can have these lab findings also, but the patient would have other symptoms such as fever, malaise, arthritis/arthralgia, and rash. Leukemia is the best answer to explain the x-ray and lab findings, the chief complaint and lack of other symptoms.

308. Answer: A

The correct answer is it would be best to give it after he has received factor replacement and then he should have direct pressure at the vaccine site for at least 2 minutes. *Haemophilus influenzae* vaccine also can be given as a subcutaneous injection in those with bleeding diathesis like hemophilia. Data indicates that the immune responses are similar in this patient population.

309. Answer: E

The correct answer is parvovirus B-19. Parvovirus in sickle cell patients has now been classically described as this case illustrates. Patients develop a red cell aplasia with no reticulocyte production. Treatment with IVIG may be beneficial. The characteristic finding in the bone marrow is GIANT pronormoblasts.

310. Answer: D

The correct answer is warfarin administration. Increased PT with a normal PTT and platelets indicates warfarin administration usually. Factor VII deficiency could do this also.

311. Answer: B

The correct answer is chronic myelogenous leukemia (CML). I know this is a "simple" knowledge question..but believe it or not they will ask you this one somewhere on the test. They are likely to give you a scenario of someone you diagnose this in and then ask you to name the chromosomal abnormality associated with this disease. So, bottom line—KNOW IT!!!!!!

312. Answer: D

The correct answer is hereditary spherocytosis. The clues here are the splenomegaly at age 15 (pretty much rules out Sickle Cell disease—remember they auto-splenectomize) and the elevated MCHC, increased osmotic fragility and the decreased red cell survival. The history of gallstones in relatives at early ages is also common in this disease. It is quite common and occurs in 1/5000 in northern Europeans.

313. Answer: A

The correct answer is Protein C deficiency. Coumarin-induced skin necrosis has been well described in patients with protein C deficiency. The skin lesions most commonly occur on the breasts, buttocks, and legs. The penis is also a described site. The theory is that an imbalance in homeostasis occurs favoring thrombosis during the early phases of coumarin administration. We know that protein C has a short half life of about 14 hours compared to some of the vitamin-K dependent factors such as factor X—and a rapid drop in the protein C concentration could produce this scenario.

314. Answer: A

The correct answer is α-thalassemia trait. This occurs when people have deletion of 2 of the 4 alpha-chain genes. These individuals tend to have a microcytic and slightly hypochromic red cell but without significant anemia or hemolysis. Hemoglobin electrophoresis can be normal or may show a decreased amount of hemoglobin A2. All of the other abnormalities listed would have microcytosis but the hemoglobin electrophoresis would be abnormal.

315. Answer: B

The correct answer is hydration and analgesia. She is having a sickle cell pain crisis that can be frequently precipitated by upper respiratory infection or dehydration. It can be very difficult to distinguish from a crisis and an acute abdomen so vigilance must be observed. Hydration is the key initially!! Hydroxyurea may reduce the incidence of sickle crises by increasing synthesis of fetal hemoglobin but has no role in an acute crisis. Antibiotics would only be administered if an infection was documented. Chest syndrome is something to be very concerned about in this patient and would require aggressive monitoring of her condition.

316. Answer: C

The correct answer is to stop PTU and schedule a follow-up appointment. She has severe neutropenia likely as an idiosyncratic reaction to PTU. She is at risk for overwhelming, life-threatening infection but at the moment without signs of fever or other signs of infection she can be followed as an outpatient. Steroids are not useful in this setting. You would never continue the offending drug. Almost always severe drug-induced neutropenia reverses fairly quickly and therefore consideration for bone marrow transplant is not indicated at this point.

317. Answer: E

The correct answer is plasmapheresis. This woman has thrombocytopenic purpura (TTP). You can put this together very easily: Hemolytic anemia with fragmented red cells, thrombocytopenia, fever, mental status changes and renal dysfunction WITHOUT evidence of disseminated intravascular coagulation (DIC) is classic for TTP. Plasmapheresis or exchange transfusion is the preferred treatment.

318. Answer: B

The correct "incorrect" answer is intravascular hemolysis has likely occurred. This presentation is consistent with a delayed transfusion reaction. Immediate transfusion reactions that would manifest as intravascular hemolysis are most commonly due to ABO incompatibility. Usually these are due to clerical error. Fever, malaise and a drop in hematocrit 1 week after red cell transfusion are typical of delayed transfusion reactions which are usually mediated by antibodies to Rh unless the patient is Rh-negative, then it is mediated by antibodies to anti-Duffy, Anti-Kell, or Anti-Kidd. These antibodies coat the donor red cells which results in a positive direct Coombs' test. Less commonly, the donor's plasma could contain antibodies that could react with the recipient's cells. WHEW! Doesn't this stuff just drive you crazy!

319. Answer: A

The correct answer is she has developed alloantibodies in her serum. Patients who receive a large number of transfusions frequently will develop a large panel of alloantibodies. This makes it difficult to type and match appropriate blood for these patients. The presence of these antibodies may or may not produce hemolysis if blood containing a potential target antigen is transfused; however, blood banks will not allow transfusion of these products unless it is an emergency situation.

320. Answer: C

The correct answer is folate in large doses can correct the megaloblastic anemia; but it does not correct the neurologic abnormalities. Antiparietal-cell antibodies are common and seen in 90% of those with pernicious anemia. Gastrin levels are usually elevated in those with pernicious anemia.

321. Answer: E

The correct answer is impaired transfer of reticuloendothelial storage iron to marrow erythroid precursors. The anemia of chronic disease is usually a normochromic, normocytic anemia. Bone marrow examination will show normal red cell maturation. Hemolysis does not usually occur. Hemoglobin synthesis is usually normal also. Patients usually have a low serum iron and a low total transferrin level. Storage iron is usually quite abundant. However, there is a decreased amount of iron in erythroblasts—this indicates a defect in the transfer of reticuloendothelial iron to immature red blood cells.

322. Answer: C

The correct answer is hemolysis is commonly induced by infection. Viruses or bacterial infection are most common and they induce an environmental oxidant stress. Drugs such as dapsone, sulfonamides, antimalarial agents and vitamin K can also trigger hemolysis. The gene for G6PD is on the X-chromosome; therefore it is a sex-linked trait. Men are more commonly involved than women. The Mediterranean variant is more severe than the A-type—found in the majority of African-Americans. The Heinz bodies can only be seen with special supravital stains. G6PD levels decrease as the red cell ages. So, during an acute episode of hemolysis, it is a bad time to check for the deficiency as a false-negative test will be seen as the newer cells being made during hemolysis will have higher levels of G6PD than older cells.

323. Answer: A

The correct answer is to check Factor VII levels. The finding of a prolonged PT and a normal PTT suggests a defect in the extrinsic coagulation cascade. Factor VII deficiency is RARE and is autosomal recessive—however, looking at the choices this is the best test to order. Remember on the Boards—go with what is the best possible answer! Factor VIII deficiency as well as the presence of coagulation factor inhibitors (Factor VIII inhibitor is the most common) would prolong the PTT. α_2–antiplasmin deficiency results in a bleeding disorder with accelerated clot lysis; the PT and PTT are normal in these patients.

324. Answer: B

The correct answer is that hemolytic uremic syndrome would be least likely to produce a thrombocytosis. Remember, it is a disease most commonly of children and results in a condition similar to thrombotic thrombocytopenic purpura! Thrombocytopenia is very common in hemolytic uremic syndrome. All of the other conditions/diseases listed would be more likely to produce a thrombocytosis.

325. Answer: B

The correct answer is aspirin. She has von Willebrand's disease and using aspirin would further aggravate her ability to aggregate platelet response. The other drugs listed are not contraindicated in von Willebrand's.

326. Answer: D

The correct answer is Factor XII deficiency. Platelet deficiency will result in normal PT and PTT except bleeding time will be abnormal. von Willebrand's will result in normal PT and PTT but an abnormally prolonged bleeding time with normal platelet aggregation. Factor VII deficiency will result in abnormal prolongation of the PT but a normal PTT. Glanzmann thrombasthenia will result in a normal PT, PTT but an abnormal bleeding time as well as abnormal platelet aggregation.

327. Answer: A

The correct answer is patients lack glycoprotein 1b. Patients have severely decreased platelet adhesion because of the lack of glycoprotein 1b. The platelets cannot bind to von Willebrand Factor. They usually have a modestly low platelet count also. It is an autosomal recessive disease.

328. Answer: D

The correct answer is it is due to a deficiency of glycoprotein IIb-IIIa complex. This is an autosomal recessive disorder. The lack of this glycoprotein complex does NOT permit fibrinogen to cross connect resulting in severe bleeding. Platelet counts are usually normal in this disease.

329. Answer: B

The correct answer is iron deficiency anemia. She has the classic symptoms and findings. Her history of menorrhagia is common and frequently results in iron deficiency anemia in younger women. The other diagnoses at her age are very unlikely. Remember common things are common and rare things are rare.

330. Answer: E

The correct answer is myelodysplastic syndrome. Myelodysplastic syndrome is UNLIKELY. It is usually seen in elderly patients (she is quite young) and is characterized by HIGH MCVs and hypercellular bone marrows. Iron deficiency anemia will give you a low MCV with anemia as she has. In the anemia of chronic disease you usually have a normal MCV but it can be low on occasion. The thalassemias (alpha and beta) will produce a microcytic anemia as she has. Sideroblastic anemia is rare but would have these findings.

331. Answer: B

The correct answer is Factor XIII deficiency. This disorder may be inherited or acquired and frequently causes severe bleeding problems. In this disorder, the bleeding time, PT and PTT are all normal!! The screening test for factor XIII deficiency is a clot solubility in urea assay. People with Factor XII and prekallikrein deficiency also have prolongation of PTT but do not have problems with surgery. Normal bleeding time excludes thrombasthenia—an inherited disorder of platelet aggregation. Protein S is a vitamin K-dependent plasma protein and a cofactor for expression of the anticoagulant activity of activated protein C.

332. Answer: A

The correct answer is that normal levels of protein C rules out the disease—this is INCORRECT!!!!!!!!!!!! Protein C is an anticoagulant which inactivates clotting factors V and VII. When deficient, it can lead to thrombosis commonly of the lower extremity deep veins as well as the iliofemoral or mesenteric veins. The majority are spontaneous while the rest occur in association with a stress such as surgery or pregnancy. It is inherited as an autosomal dominant disease. Two forms of the disease exist: 1) normal levels of protein C, but they are a biologically dysfunctional protein, and 2) deficient levels. Therefore, just measuring the level of protein C will not "rule out" the disease. You must also measure "tests of function". Besides the inherited form, acquired protein C deficiency can occur. This can happen with DIC, severe liver disease, nephrotic syndrome, etc.

333. Answer: C

The correct answer is iron deficiency anemia. With a microcytic anemia and a HIGH RDW think of iron deficiency anemia.

334. Answer: B

The correct "incorrect" answer is Thromboasthenia (Glanzmann's syndrome). The congenital bilateral absence of radius is also known as "Thrombocytopenia absent radius syndrome" or TAR. Glanzmann's thrombasthenia is an autosomal recessive disorder characterized by normal platelet numbers but don't function properly. Thus they have a bleeding disorder because of poor function, not lack of numbers.

335. Answer: C

The correct answer is idiopathic thrombocytopenia purpura (ITP). It is usually preceded by a viral illness and is caused by antibody-mediated destruction of platelets. Acute ITP mainly occurs between 2 and 5 years. Chronic ITP is more common in children age 7 to 10 years. Clinical features include abrupt onset of bleeding with common sites being dermal/mucosal and absence of hepatosplenomegaly and lymphadenopathy. Lab reveals isolated low platelet count with normal hemoglobin and MCV. Peripheral blood smear is normal except for low platelet count. Bone marrow (which would show normal to increased number of megakaryocytes) is usually not needed unless corticosteroid therapy is initiated and sometimes not even then. If the patient has stable hemoglobin with no active bleeding other than purpura, no therapy is needed because the spontaneous remission rate is high. For active bleeding, the patient would need therapy which could include corticosteroids, IV gamma globulin, and/or anti-D immune globulin.

336. Answer: A

The correct answer is bone marrow shows decreased number of megakaryocytes. This patient has Kasabach-Merritt syndrome that consists of a large hemangioma (or kaposiform hemangioendothelioma) with localized intravascular coagulation within the vascular lesion causing thrombocytopenia and hypofibrinogenemia. The bone marrow shows normal or increased number of megakaryocytes. Treatment includes systemic steroids, embolization, cyclophosphamide, radiation therapy, and antifibrinolytic therapy.

337. Answer: A

The correct "incorrect" answer is children with retinoblastoma confined to the retina have a poor survival rate. Retinoblastoma is the most common intraocular tumor in childhood. It is of neuroectodermal origin arising from embryonic retinal cells. It does have both inheritable and non-inheritable forms. The inheritable form is caused by a mutation in the retinoblastoma gene which is a tumor suppressor gene.

Most patients present with leukocoria (60%). Sometimes asymmetry of the affected eye is noted. Strabismus occurs in 20% (if macula is involved).

Evaluation consists of an ophthalmologic exam under anesthesia. A CT scan is needed to evaluate the optic nerve and extension of tumor. A bone marrow aspirate with CSF cytology can evaluate metastatic disease.

Radiation therapy is used for all patients, but chemotherapy is added for those with metastatic disease. Children with retinoblastoma confined to the retina have a >90% 5-year survival rate. Those with disease involving the optic nerve past the lamina cribrosa have a 5-year survival rate of 40%, and those with metastatic disease rarely survive. Patients with the inheritable form have increased risk of developing other tumors.

338. Answer: D

The correct answer is osteosarcoma. This is the most common primary bone tumor in childhood usually occurring in adolescence. Long tubular bones are usually affected. Patients present with deep bone pain (sometimes waking them at night), palpable mass, and x-ray findings (the classic appearance is the sunburst pattern). Biopsy of the lesion is needed to confirm the diagnosis. A work-up looking for metastatic disease includes chest CT and bone scan. Treatment consists of chemotherapy before and after surgery resection. Patients with nonmetastatic extremity involvement have up to 75% cure rate. 20-30% with limited lung metastases can also be cured. Those with other metastatic involvement have poor prognosis.

339. Answer: C

The correct answer is the tumor is radiosensitive. The peak incidence is in the 1st decade usually between the ages of 3 and 5. Obstruction of the ventricular system occurs commonly and early—which results in papilledema early. The prognosis is poor for this tumor even though it is radiosensitive—mainly because the tumor has usually spread to the meninges already.

340. Answer: E

The correct "incorrect" answer is Hodgkin's lymphoma. This most commonly occurs in older children and adolescents. Leukemia is borderline but more commonly occurs between the ages of 2 and 6. All of the others occur in children in the first few years of life.

341. Answer: B

The correct answer is Wilm's tumor. The syndrome of Wilm's and aniridia is known as Miller's or aniridia-Wilm's tumor syndrome. Children with aniridia should be followed closely with physical as well as ultrasound abdominal exams during the first few years of life. If the aniridia is due to an autosomal dominant or recessive form of inheritance (as opposed to sporadic) then they do not require such follow-up. It appears only the sporadic form is at risk for Wilm's tumor.

342. Answer: C

The correct answer is to remove the central venous catheter and start empiric broad-spectrum antibiotics as well as amphotericin B. In this severely neutropenic patient, as well as because of her overwhelmingly immunocompromised state from her recent transplant and medications, all bacterial etiologies, as well as severe fungemias, must be considered particularly with *Candida* species. Therefore, it is reasonable to start broad-spectrum antibiotics as well as amphotericin B initially. The line must be removed at any sign of infection particularly if fungal infection is suspected. Note, this is different from the general febrile neutropenic patient without a source! She has a probable source--her line, and you need to treat aggressively!

343. Answer: B

The correct answer is that a change in the color of the lesion warrants further workup for potential malignancy. One of the characteristics that distinguish a superficial spreading malignant melanoma from a normal mole is a change in the color of the lesion. Another warning sign is if the border becomes irregular. Usually the first change noted is a "darkening" in color or a change in the borders of the lesion. Excisional biopsy should be done promptly because early diagnosis and excision reduce mortality.

344. Answer: A

The correct answer is cystic fibrosis. Cystic fibrosis (CF) is NOT associated with development of malignancy. Fanconi's anemia is associated with cytogenetic abnormalities and has an increased risk of cancer. Approximately 10% of patients with neurofibromatosis develop sarcomatous changes. Ataxia-telangiectasia is associated with lymphoma. Familial polyposis coli predisposes to colon cancer in all patients with this disorder.

345. Answer: A

The correct "incorrect" answer is anthracycline agents suppress bone marrow stem cells to a greater degree than they do more "committed" hematopoietic cells. This is a false statement. The anthracycline agents generally suppress the more "committed" cells instead of the stem cell lines. The other statements are correct. Cisplatin causes large renal losses of potassium and magnesium that in turn leads to hypocalcemia. Vincristine is a relatively mild myelosuppressive agent and can be used in periods of low white blood cell counts.

346. Answer: B

The correct answer is ovarian cancer of germ cell lineage. Most ovarian cancers are of epithelial cell lineage however she had evidence of hormonal abnormalities with the hirsutism, deepening voice, and clitorimegaly. All of these findings are consistent with virilization and androgen production. These ovarian germ cell tumors can be treated similarly to testicular carcinoma in men and respond to therapy with cisplatin and etoposide.

347. Answer: D

The correct answer is he has entered an accelerated or blastic phase. The Philadelphia chromosome is the diagnostic "hallmark" of chronic myeloid leukemia. Remember that it involves the translocation between chromosome 22 and chromosome 9. Older patients with CML usually have a chronic benign phase for 3-4 years. The most commonly observed cytogenetic event to signify an accelerated or blast phase is duplication of the Philadelphia chromosome!

348. Answer: E

The correct answer is early onset coronary artery disease. Within months of mantle irradiation, about 15% develop LOWER extremity paresthesia upon flexion of the neck, also known as Lhermitte's sign. Radiation pneumonitis is also a concern in a small percentage of patients (<5%). Other complications of mantle radiation include pericardial effusion, myocardial injury and an increased risk of coronary artery disease. Hypothyroidism occurs in over 80% of patients! Breast cancer and lung cancer are increased in incidence as well as stomach, skin and soft tissue sarcomas. Acute leukemias are rare in patients not treated with chemotherapy agents.

349. Answer: A

The correct answer is biopsy. Cervical cancer mortality is so preventable because it is easily revealed by the Pap smear. But it's only a screening test. If the Pap returns with low-grade squamous intraepithelial lesion (or high-grade) then a punch biopsy is required for diagnosis of CIN or invasive carcinoma. If the biopsy then shows CIN I (slight dysplasia) this may resolve, and does not require treatment. Follow-up with a repeat Pap smear in 4-6 months. CIN II and III (moderate and severe dysplasia) are treated with ablative therapy, either cryotherapy or laser. If the punch biopsy returns showing invasive carcinoma, staging is done, and the patient is treated with hysterectomy or radiation, or both. If the biopsy did not make the stage of the pre malignancy clear, then conization is indicated.

350. Answer: A

The correct answer is seminoma. Seminomas comprise 60% of germ cell tumors, and non-seminomas the remaining 40%. Germ cell tumors comprise 95% of all testicular tumors. Sertoli cell cancer is uncommon. Torsion is an acute process accompanied by intense pain and tenderness. Hydroceles are cystic, not solid or firm.

351. Answer: D

The correct answer is acute myelogenous leukemia (AML). AML is unusual in that lymphadenopathy is NOT common. Splenomegaly also is NOT common in AML.

352. Answer: B

The correct answer is neurotoxicity. These patients can develop a peripheral neuropathy.

353. Answer: B

The correct answer is proceed with combination chemotherapy without laparotomy. This patient has Stage IIIB Hodgkin's disease. Further workup is not needed as the CT scan indicated disease on both sides of the diaphragm. Additionally he has "B" symptoms with night sweats. Treatment should proceed with combination chemotherapy. Further surgery or workup is not indicated at this time.

354. Answer: B

The correct answer is if the genital warts are due to Human Papillomavirus type 16 or 18. The way I remember this is that kids get their driver's license in most states at age 16 and can vote at age 18— (both of these are potentially bad things depending on the habits of the 16 and 18 year old). These types are thought to express an E7 protein which binds to the retinoblastoma protein inactivating the retinoblastoma tumor-suppressor gene. Types 31 and 35 have also been implicated. I don't have any good pneumonics for 31 and 35 except that some view 31 as a "bad age" as you are now in your 30s for sure and 35 is really bad cause you are ½ way to 40. (sorry not much help on these 2).

355. Answer: D

The correct answer is 95%. With a seminoma and confined to the testes (Stage I) there is a 95% survival rate with radiation therapy. This is one of the most curable types of cancer especially if treated and recognized early.

356. Answer: A

The correct answer is ovarian cancer. Not a lot of explanation here—sorry. This is pretty straightforward just memorize it.

357. Answer: D

The correct answer is age of diagnosis. Children under 1 year of age do markedly better than those over 1 year of age. The prognosis is poor for children older than a year of age. Neuroblastoma can present in many different ways so be on the look out for it on the test. They will try and get you to figure out if it is Wilm's tumor or neuroblastoma. Remember that neuroblastoma produces all sorts of biologic substances including catecholamines, ferritin, and neuron-specific enolase.

358. Answer: C

The correct "incorrect" answer is the tumors usually present late in life. Usually they present early life and commonly are seen at birth. The rest of the listed elements are true.

359. Answer: D

The correct answer is microscopy would show diffuse increase in mesangial cells and matrix. This patient has the features of nephrotic syndrome including proteinuria, edema, hypoalbuminemia, and hyperlipidemia. Minimal change nephrotic syndrome (MCNS) is the most common nephrotic syndrome of childhood (especially ages 2-6 years old) and 95% of these children respond to steroid therapy. If this patient had not responded to steroids, a renal biopsy would be necessary to rule out other causes of nephrotic syndrome. The etiology of MCNS is unknown and light microscopy is normal. Electron microscopy shows only foot process fusion.

Complement C3 is normal or slightly elevated in MCNS whereas it is decreased in other causes of nephrotic syndrome (i.e. membranoproliferative glomerulonephritis or postinfectious glomerulonephritis). The serum calcium is decreased due to reduction in the albumin-bound fraction. These patients are at increased risk for peritonitis (usually pneumococcal and should therefore get this vaccine) because of the presence of ascitic fluid and decreased resistance of infection.

Occasional treatment with albumin and diuretics may be needed for severe edema and ascites. Most children have repeated relapses until spontaneous resolution of disease when the patient reaches their late twenties.

360. Answer: A

The correct answer is immediately refer him to a pediatric dialysis unit. This patient has hemolytic uremic syndrome (HUS) which usually follows the onset of diarrhea (most commonly caused by *E.coli* 0157:H7 or *Shigella*) by 3-14 days. HUS presents with the sudden onset of pallor, irritability, lethargy, and oliguria. Edema, petechiae, and hepatosplenomegaly may also be present.

Lab reveals elevated urea and creatinine, hemolytic anemia, and thrombocytopenia. Blood smear shows helmet cells, burr cells, and fragmented RBCs. Coombs is negative. PT/PTT are normal. Urine abnormalities are mild with low-grade proteinuria and hematuria.

Early and frequent dialysis is needed for patients with HUS and renal failure. Although this patient may eventually need blood products, you should first get him to a dialysis center. Dialysis, in addition to medical management of the hematologic and renal manifestations, results in more than 90% of patients surviving the acute phase. The majority of these will regain normal renal function. Long-term follow-up is needed to watch for development of hypertension or chronic kidney disease.

361. Answer: B

The correct answer is this will likely give erroneously high readings. The bladder of the cuff should cover at least two-thirds of the length of the arm and should wrap around at least ¾ of the circumference. A cuff covering only ½ of the length of the upper arm is likely to give too high of a reading.

362. Answer: D

The correct "incorrect" answer is responsible for increased renin in hypertensive subjects. Converting enzyme inhibitors are effective antihypertensive agents, with rare side effects of cough (10%), reversible renal insufficiency, hyperkalemia and angioedema (<0.1%). They have been proven effective in slowing the rate of progression of diabetic and other proteinuric renal diseases. Discontinuation rates for hyperkalemia are low (<1% in studies). Patients with renal artery stenosis often have an exaggerated response to converting enzyme inhibitors. Renin levels are high in patients taking these agents.

363. Answer: B

The correct answer is her total body sodium is approximately normal. In a hyponatremic patient, low urine osmolality always diagnoses psychogenic polydipsia. Treatment is supportive and while hypertonic saline should be considered in symptomatic patients with hyponatremia, this hyponatremia will likely resolve at a rapid rate with fluid restriction alone. In fact, if chronic, water therapy is sometimes needed to keep the rate of correction at <2mEq/l/hour. Diuretic abuse will lead to a higher urine osmolality when not in use or a higher urine sodium when in use. High ADH levels lead to a concentrated urine. While the patient's volume status is mildly expanded from water, total body sodium is regulated normally and kept negligibly lower than normal.

364. Answer: D

The correct answer is alkalinization of the urine. Rhabdomyolysis classically presents as acute renal failure with pigment in the urine in excess of red blood cells, muddy brown casts and disproportionate increases in creatinine compared to BUN. Alcohol and cocaine use are often precipitating factors. Treatment includes optimization of volume status and a forced, alkaline diuresis, if possible. No indications for dialysis have arisen, the hypocalcemia (or hyperkalemia) does not warrant emergent therapy as intracellular stores may be released later and the high phosphorus is also a cause for hypocalcemia that should not be treated aggressively with calcium (may precipitate metastatic calcification). The patient is hyponatremic and does not need free water replacement at this time.

365. Answer: A

The correct answer is low calcium diet. Stone formation in a patient with hypokalemia, an anion gap acidosis with a high urine pH, a positive urine anion gap, and a family history of stones suggests Type I RTA (distal). Abnormal growth may also be seen. Bicarbonate or citrate therapy corrects the acidosis and citrate corrects the associated hypocitraturia; fluid therapy helps prevent stones. Thiazide therapy might help limit stone formation but might exacerbate hypokalemia. Low calcium diets are of no value in this setting.

366. Answer: E

The correct answer is renal artery stenosis. Alkalosis is generated when acid is lost or excess bicarbonate is generated in the kidney. It is then maintained by ongoing proximal reclamation and distal acidification driven by aldosterone. Chloride depletion contributes in vomiting, contraction, prior diuretic use and is diagnosed by a low urine chloride (<10 mEq/L). Severe hypokalemia can lead to a chloride-resistant alkalosis but this is more commonly seen with hyper-aldosterone states such as renal artery stenosis, licorice intake or primary hyperaldosteronism.

367. Answer: A

The correct "incorrect" answer is cause hypercalcemia in some users. Loop diuretics inhibit the Na, K 2 Cl transporter leading to natriuresis, kaliuresis and reduction in blood pressure. They enhance proximal sodium reabsorption leading to alkalosis and increases in uric acid, occasionally precipitating gout. They are associated with calcium and magnesium losses, and are used in the treatment of significant hypercalcemia.

368. Answer: C

The correct answer is can cause acute and chronic renal damage by means of vasoconstriction. Cyclosporine works by inhibiting T cell function, inhibiting production of interleukin-2. It does not cause pancytopenia. There are multiple drug interactions to be concerned with and toxicities include renal dysfunction due to vasoconstriction, hypertension, hyperkalemia, gout hirsutism, neurotoxicity and infection. However, the incidence of infection in cyclosporine-treated patients is no greater than that of patients taking azathioprine and steroids as their immunosuppression.

369. Answer: D

The correct answer is enalapril. Multiple studies have demonstrated reduction in proteinuria with ACE inhibitors and increasing studies are demonstrating enhanced renal survival as well as enhanced cardiac survival with these agents. A biopsy is generally unrewarding as the specificity of a diagnosis of diabetic nephropathy approaches 100% when patients have proteinuric renal insufficiency and retinopathy. Renal artery stenosis is unlikely in this case. Dihydropyridines appear inferior to ACEI in studies and may exacerbate proteinuria. Weight loss, sugar control and low salt diet are reasonable but are not the mainstay of therapy.

370. Answer: C

The correct answer is acute renal failure secondary to rhabdomyolysis associated with hypophosphatemia. This patient has alcoholic ketoacidosis (AKA) and presents with the classic constellation of findings of alcohol binging, hypoglycemia and an anion gap metabolic acidosis. These patients usually have hypophosphatemia, which can be severe, and hypomagnesemia. The hypophosphatemia can be severe enough to result in rhabdomyolysis. The diagnosis of alcoholic ketoacidosis may be missed as these patients improve quickly with glucose administration and the ketones are initially beta-hydroxybutyrate and are not detected in the serum until they are converted to acetoacetate. Recognition of the clinical syndrome allows one to monitor and appropriately replace phosphorus early in the hospitalization to prevent complications such as rhabdomyolysis.

Note that acute renal failure secondary to ethylene glycol intoxication is incorrect. The most important clue to the diagnosis of either ethylene glycol or methanol intoxication is an osmolar gap greater than 10. The osmolality is calculated as 2 x sodium + glucose/18+ BUN/2.8. This value will be significantly greater than the measured osmolality in patients with alcohol, methanol or ethylene glycol ingestion. Also in patients with ethylene glycol ingestion, calcium oxalate crystals may be present in the urine, a rather important clue on Board exams. Treatment includes ethanol administration, thiamine, and pyridoxine.

For the answer of methanol intoxication, an osmolar gap is usually present along with an anion gap acidosis. These patients typically present with a fruity odor and blurred vision due to the degradation of methanol to formaldehyde and formic acid, which is toxic to the optic nerve. Treatment includes ethanol administration and hemodialysis.

Isopropyl alcohol is metabolized to acetone and may result in ketosis; however, these patients do not have an acidosis.

The diagnosis of hepatorenal syndrome should be suspected in patients with cirrhosis, portal hypertension and ascites. Patients who develop acute renal failure in this setting must be evaluated for intravascular volume depletion, frequently associated with diuretics, vomiting or bleeding or they may develop acute renal failure associated with acute tubular necrosis associated with many of the medications they receive. The diagnosis of HRS depends on demonstrating a benign urinalysis, extremely low fractional excretion of sodium, no response to volume repletion, and exclusion of obstruction or toxic causes.

371. Answer: B

The correct answer is urine eosinophils--In hospitalized patients who develop acute renal failure, one must always consider medications as the cause. In this patient, the administration of trimethoprim/sulfamethoxazole should raise the possibility of acute interstitial nephritis. Acute interstitial nephritis is a hypersensitivity reaction, which frequently produces eosinophilia in the serum and eosinophils in the urine; however, patients may still have AIN even in the absence of this finding. More recently, Hansel stain has been shown to be most effective in demonstrating eosinophils, though Wright stain has traditionally been used. The most common medications that cause acute interstitial nephritis are the non-steroidal anti-inflammatory drugs, and antibiotics including sulfa-based antibiotics, cephalosporins, quinolones, and penicillins.

To ultrasound the kidney is incorrect – An appropriate diagnostic study which should be ordered to exclude obstruction. In this young patient, without underlying reason for obstruction to occur, this is unlikely to be abnormal. Particularly in older men, both urinary catheterization for evidence of post-void residual and ultrasound are more likely to demonstrate evidence of obstructive uropathy.

A 24-hour urine for protein and creatinine clearance is incorrect– in the setting of acute renal failure, the creatinine clearance cannot be accurately determined as the creatinine is constantly rising indicating the patient must have markedly diminished GFR. In the absence of significant proteinuria, the 24-hour urine is unlikely to add further information in this patient.

A Urine electrophoresis is not correct – this is the appropriate diagnostic study to order when one suspects light chains (Bence Jones Protein) may be present in the urine. This is particularly important when evaluating patients for either multiple myeloma or amyloidosis—both diseases much more common in adults. Amyloidosis is typically associated with nephrotic syndrome, not present in this patient and amyloid of the kidney is usually also found when patients with myeloma also have nephrotic syndrome.

An ANCA is not appropriate. – antineutrophilic cytoplasmic antibody is a useful diagnostic study in the evaluation of acute glomerulonephritis, particularly when either microscopic polyarteritis or Wegener's granulomatosis is suspected. This patient however has no significant hematuria or proteinuria, therefore making the diagnosis of acute glomerulonephritis most unlikely. While the ANCA may be very helpful in cases of rapidly progressive glomerulonephritis, it is not as helpful in the diagnosis of other forms of renal disease.

372. Answer: D

The correct answer is this patient is not likely to develop progressive renal failure – the most likely diagnosis in the acute onset of severe nephrotic syndrome, particularly in a younger patient, is minimal change disease. The initial treatment is corticosteroid therapy. Most patients will respond to treatment with prednisone alone. Patients who relapse after prednisone therapy should be retreated but frequent relapsers may also require cytotoxic therapy. In contrast to other types of glomerular disease, minimal change disease is not a progressive form of renal failure and the long term prognosis is excellent.

It is incorrect to choose treatment that is initiated with steroids and cytotoxic therapy to prevent progressive renal disease – initial therapy of minimal change disease is with prednisone alone with cytotoxic therapy being added only for patients who frequently relapse or in whom remission cannot be achieved.

An unlikely diagnosis is focal and segmental glomerulosclerosis. FSGS presents with a more insidious onset and is more commonly associated with both hypertension and impairment of renal function. Particularly in young African-American adults, presentation with idiopathic nephrotic syndrome, hypertension and progressive renal failure strongly suggests the diagnosis of FSGS. FSGS is also treated with prednisone initially with those patients achieving remission having a significantly better prognosis.

Another incorrect choice would be treatment initiated with Cyclosporine-- while cyclosporine has been used for treatment of steroid-resistant minimal change disease in children; it is not considered initial therapy.

Finally, ACE-Inhibitor therapy should be used in patients with heavy proteinuria. ACE-inhibitors exert an important anti-proteinuric affect and should be used in patients with hypertension and proteinuria. However they may also be an important adjunct to therapy in patients with heavy proteinuria even with normotension.

373. Answer: A

The correct answer is to order complement levels. The presence of RBC casts establishes the diagnosis of glomerulonephritis, therefore complete serologic studies to exclude secondary causes is essential. The most likely diagnosis in a patient with gross hematuria immediately following an upper respiratory infection is IgA nephropathy. While the diagnosis can only be established by renal biopsy, complement levels and hepatitis studies must be performed to exclude underlying secondary causes, such as lupus, post-infectious glomerulonephritis, or HCV-associated GN.

Referral to a urologist is incorrect – it is essential, in patients with hematuria, to determine whether the bleeding is most likely coming from the upper or lower tract. Clues to the diagnosis of upper tract bleeding include the presence of red blood cell casts, proteinuria associated with hematuria, and dysmorphic red blood cells. In patients with isolated hematuria where none of these features are present, urologic evaluation would be appropriate, particularly in older patients where the diagnosis of GU malignancy must be excluded. This patient has glomerulonephritis based on the RBC casts and urologic referral would only delay diagnosis.

Immediate referral for renal biopsy is incorrect – patients who present with evidence of glomerulonephritis will usually require renal biopsy to establish a diagnosis. Of particular concern are those patients with acute glomerulonephritis as manifested by evidence of salt and water retention with renal insufficiency. Patients with rapidly progressive glomerulonephritis in which renal function can deteriorate even on a daily basis, should always be evaluated for urgent renal biopsy to quickly establish a diagnosis and initiate appropriate therapy. In this patient, outpatient evaluation should be performed before biopsy is performed.

It is incorrect to begin prednisone 60 mg daily – patients with IgA nephropathy and normal renal function, especially without proteinuria, require no therapy. Of greater concern are patients with progressive disease who are likely to have significant proteinuria. More recent studies have evaluated the use of both steroid and cytotoxic therapy in patients with proteinuria and progressive renal disease with data suggesting these treatments may be of benefit. This would not be appropriate in this patient.

Hearing evaluation is not indicated – one of the considerations in younger patients who present with hematuria due to glomerulonephritis is Alport's Syndrome, (hereditary nephritis). The hallmarks of this disorder are hearing loss and glomerulonephritis, occasionally with associated ocular abnormalities. This disease is typically expressed much more severely in men than in women. While the family history can be very suggestive, the diagnosis can only be established with certainty by renal biopsy demonstrating particular thinning or lamellation of the glomerular basement membrane seen on electron microscopy.

374. Answer: A

The correct answer is metabolic acidosis, respiratory alkalosis, and metabolic alkalosis – while it is apparent that this patient has diabetic ketoacidosis, it may not be apparent that she has a triple acid base disorder. In evaluating all patients with electrolyte and acid base disorders, the anion gap must also be calculated. In this patient, the anion gap is 32, which is consistent with her anion gap metabolic acidosis associated with diabetic ketoacidosis. When one calculates what the PCO2 should be for a patient with metabolic acidosis with a serum bicarbonate of 12 (1.5 x HCO3 + 8), that value is 26. This patient's PCO2 is 20 so she is therefore overventilating and therefore must also have a respiratory alkalosis. Finally, one can also calculate the "delta anion gap", which is the amount of bicarbonate that has been consumed to raise the anion gap from the normal value of 12 to 32 in this patient, which is 20. Since the patient consumed 20 millimoles of bicarbonate per liter and her current serum bicarbonate is 12, then she must have had an "initial" bicarbonate of 32 (20 + 12 = 32). This therefore uncovers the hidden metabolic alkalosis, which one would expect in a patient with severe vomiting. Appropriate therapy is still fluid resuscitation and insulin administration, while watching for the development of hypokalemia.

375. Answer: D

The correct answer is Bartter's syndrome – In evaluating metabolic alkalosis, it is extremely helpful to order urine chloride, which will be elevated when the alkalosis is due to both endogenous and exogenous steroid excess or due to Bartter's Syndrome. Bartter's syndrome is caused by a mutation of the Na-K 2-chloride transporter in the thick ascending limb of Henle. Bartter's Syndrome is a familial disorder characterized by metabolic alkalosis, normotension, normokalemia, hypomagnesemia and elevated renin and aldosterone levels.

Liddle's Syndrome is incorrect – this familial disorder is characterized by hypertension, hypokalemia and low renin and aldosterone. It is caused by a defect in the collecting duct sodium channel. Amiloride is the appropriate treatment.

Primary hyperaldosteronism is incorrect – These patients present with hypertension, hypokalemia and metabolic alkalosis. Renin levels are low while aldosterone levels are high and non-suppressible. Primary hyperaldosteronism is due to either unilateral adrenal adenoma or bilateral adrenal hyperplasia.

Addison's Disease is incorrect – patients with Addison's Disease have mineralocorticoid deficiency and therefore are normotensive or hypotensive with hyperkalemia and a metabolic acidosis.

Renal artery stenosis is incorrect – patients with renal artery stenosis may be hypokalemic with a metabolic alkalosis, but they are hypertensive. These patients have secondary hyperaldosteronism and therefore renin levels are also elevated.

376. Answer: A

The correct answer is Type I distal RTA: This patient has a non anion gap metabolic acidosis. The initial approach in NAG metabolic acidosis is to measure the urinary anion gap. This serves as a measure of urinary acidification. Normally the urine anion gap (Urine Na + K – Cl) is negative. However, in patients with urinary acidification defects, this value will be positive. Normally one should be able to acidify the urine in the face of metabolic acidosis. In this pt, the urine pH is 7 because he cannot secrete H+ ions across the concentration gradient in the distal tubule. These patients cannot lower their urine pH below 6.0 regardless of degree of acidosis. These patients also have hypercalciuria, and may develop nephrolithiasis and nephrocalcinosis. Congenital, familial RTA is associated with hearing loss--acquired Type I RTA is seen with several underlying disorders including hyperparathyroidism, and hypergammaglobulinemia. Treatment includes bicarbonate and potassium administration.

Type II RTA is incorrect: These patients typically "waste" bicarbonate, and therefore the urine pH is also high initially, along with a non-anion gap metabolic acidosis. Eventually patients have no more HCO_3 to waste and the urine pH becomes more acid. Proximal RTA may also be associated with Fanconi Syndrome and urinary loss of glucose, phosphorus, uric acid and amino acids. This disorder is not associated with nephrolithiasis or hearing loss. Important causes of acquired Type II RTA include multiple myeloma and heavy metals. These patients may require large amounts of bicarbonate administration to correct the acidosis.

Type IV RTA is incorrect: Type IV RTA is a hyperkalemic, distal RTA, most commonly occurring in diabetics, but also associated with obstructive uropathy, and other forms of tubulointerstitial renal disease. It is most often caused by aldosterone deficiency. Treatment includes sodium bicarbonate administration, fludrocortisone, and/or furosemide.

Chronic diarrhea is not a correct choice- chronic diarrhea and HCO_3 loss may cause a non-anion gap metabolic acidosis. However, urinary acidification is normal, therefore the urinary anion gap will be negative.

Salicylate intoxification is not likely- salicylate intoxification causes an anion gap metabolic acidosis and is not associated with hypokalemia. Patients typically also have a respiratory alkalosis, which serves as another clue to the diagnosis.

377. Answer: E

The correct answer is begin hydrochlorothiazide 25 mg/day. This patient most likely has congenital nephrogenic diabetes insipidus. He has thirst and polyuria. His serum sodium is borderline elevated with a relatively low urine osmolality. Neither serum nor urine suggest diabetes mellitus as a cause of his polyuria. He had a childhood history of enuresis and has never presented for medical attention. Most patients with nephrogenic diabetes insipidus learn to live with their polyuria and do not consider themselves "ill". The only treatment for nephrogenic diabetes insipidus of unknown etiology is hydrochlorothiazide as thiazide diuretics enhance distal tubule water reabsorption. The lifelong history of polyuria and the ability to concentrate the urine to near 300 mOsm/kg suggests that he does not have central diabetes insipidus, so neither vasopressin tannate in oil nor DDAVP would be effective. Water restriction would result in further hypernatremia. Although it may stimulate his kidneys to concentrate his urine somewhat more than they presently are, it would not be adequate to maintain a reasonable serum osmolality. The patient's relative hypernatremia argues strongly against a diagnosis of psychogenic polydipsia.

378. Answer: B

The correct answer is dipsticks only detect negatively charged proteins like albumin. Immunoglobulins (which is likely what he is excreting) are positively charged and therefore are not picked up on the dipstick.

379. Answer: D

The correct answer is nephrogenic diabetes insipidus. Failure to concentrate urine in the face of substantial hypertonic dehydration suggests diabetes insipidus. A nephrogenic origin is suspected when there is no increase in urine concentration after exogenous vasopressin.

380. Answer: A

The correct answer is Na 143, K 4.8, Cl-100, HCO3-10, Serum Creatinine 3.5, Arterial pH 7.25. Ethylene glycol ingestion causes acute renal failure and leads to rapid accumulation of metabolic acids. Acidosis is proportionate to the degree of renal insufficiency and is characterized by a HIGH anion gap (here AG = 33).

381. Answer: C

The correct answer is Na 140, K 2.6, Cl-115, HCO3-13, Serum Creatinine 1.9, Arterial pH 7.31, and urine pH 6.2. Amphotericin B also causes renal insufficiency with a disproportionate metabolic acidosis. However, the acidosis is due to a distal tubular acidification defect and is characterized by hyperchloremia, a normal anion gap, and inability to lower the urine pH.

382. Answer: B

The correct answer is Na 136, K 5.2, Cl-102, HCO3-20, Serum Creatinine 3.5, Arterial pH 7.36, urine pH 5.0. With a moderate glomerulonephritis, metabolic acidosis is usually mild and the anion gap is only slightly elevated, if at all.

383. Answer: A

The correct answer is Na 140, K 6.2, Cl-109, HCO3-20, Serum Creatinine 3.5, Arterial pH 7.36 urine pH 5.0. This illustrates moderate renal insufficiency with disproportionate hyperkalemia and hyperchloremic acidosis. One of the most common things to do this is diabetic nephropathy.

384. Answer: B

The correct answer is hypercalciuria. For some reason, this is found in a significant number of children with otherwise unexplained hematuria. The hematuria is not associated with stone formation. The serum level of calcium is normal.

385. Answer: E

The correct answer is it can occur with a normal urinalysis. Renal biopsies of "asymptomatic family members" of the index case have shown evidence of poststreptococcal glomerulonephritis without evidence of abnormality on urinalysis. It is more common in children between the ages of 5 and 10 years of age. It usually follows a streptococcal infection by 1 to 2 WEEKS. Usually complement levels will be low and the best treatment is observation—most will improve on their own without specific therapy.

386. Answer: E

The correct answer is all of the choices can cause nephrotic syndrome in children. Most however are usually due to minimal change disease or other underlying renal disorders.

387. Answer: D

The correct answer is it is associated with renal deposition of immunoglobulins. FSGS does not respond to steroids well and has a very poor prognosis. It ultimately leads to renal failure.

388. Answer: A

The correct answer is referral for rigid bronchoscopy. This patient had a sudden onset of cough and is at the perfect age for foreign body aspiration. The patient has unilateral wheezing and asymmetric breath sounds. CXR shows obstructive hyperinflation which is the most common finding in acute foreign body aspiration. Most foreign bodies are not radiopaque. The procedure of choice is rigid bronchoscopy when foreign body aspiration is suspected.

389. Answer: A

The correct answer is place the PPD today and give her MMR today. Simultaneous placing of PPD and administering the MMR will not affect tuberculin activity. However, giving the MMR will suppress the ability to respond to tuberculin in a week or so and will persist for 4-6 weeks. So, if they cannot be given at the same time it is best to wait 6 weeks before placing the PPD after the MMR. In this case, she needs protection against the constituents of MMR and she needs a PPD today—she should not wait for 6 weeks. So, the correct answer is to do both today. If for some reason she had received her MMR last week—then you would wait a total of 4-6 weeks before placing her PPD.

390. Answer: C

The correct answer is blastomycosis. The combination of lung mass, draining cutaneous lesion, and the finding of budding yeast should point you toward either Blastomycosis or Coccidioidomycosis. Geography will narrow down this to blastomycosis. Histoplasmosis will not usually cause skin lesions as are seen with blastomycosis or coccidioidomycosis. Treatment would be generally with oral itraconazole for about 6 months. If she was severely ill, you would use amphotericin B.

391. Answer: D

The correct answer is to order a sweat chloride test. Cystic Fibrosis may present with widely variable involvement of many organs including the lungs, pancreas, and liver. In addition, an array of signs and symptoms may occur including failure to thrive, meconium ileus, acid-base abnormalities, rectal prolapse, nasal polyps, and sinus disease. This patient's failure to thrive and recurrent respiratory infections have been difficult to track due to the frequent change in physicians. His wheezing is related to the obstructive lung disease caused by the cystic fibrosis. The stool changes are consistent with the pancreatic insufficiency from CF. Patients with CF should be developmentally normal. The split S2 with the loud pulmonary valve component is consistent with pulmonary hypertension related to the chronic respiratory disease. Liver disease associated with CF is associated with an enlarged, smooth liver with elevated transaminases. Patients with CF may have some degree of malabsorption that may contribute to an iron deficient anemia. This patient needs a sweat chloride test. Simple reassurance will further delay diagnosis. An ultrasound of the liver may need to eventually be done, but the underlying diagnosis needs to be addressed first. Recurrent pneumonias can be associated with immunoglobulin deficiencies, but the other constellation of symptoms makes CF more likely.

392. Answer: D

The correct answer is to order bronchodilators, chest physiotherapy, and DNAse. Initiation of supportive therapy should begin as soon as the diagnosis of CF is made. Aerosol therapy is used to deliver saline and bronchodilators to the lower respiratory tract. Beta-agonist, and in some instances cromolyn sodium are used in patients with bronchoconstriction. Aerosolized DNAse can improve pulmonary function and decrease pulmonary exacerbations. Chest physical therapy that includes percussion and postural drainage allows the clearance of secretions from the small airways. Chest PT should be administered 1-4 times daily, depending on lung function. Intravenous antibiotics should be administered at the first sign of infection. In some cases, inhaled tobramycin is used to suppress infection.

393. Answer: E

The correct answer is down regulation of beta-adrenergic receptors. Inhaled glucocorticoids actually cause up regulation of beta-adrenergic receptors. At one time their use was limited to patients with moderate to severe asthma, but now they are recommended as first-line agents for those with mild persistent asthma. Clinically significant adverse reactions are unlikely with appropriate pediatric doses.

394. Answer: B

The correct answer is add daily inhaled corticosteroids. This patient has mild persistent asthma and therefore requires a long-term control medication. Inhaled glucocorticoids are now considered the first-line agent for mild persistent asthma. They are safe when used at the appropriate pediatric doses. There is a delayed onset of action and therefore must be given daily. The goal will be to limit major exacerbations and the need for oral steroids.

395. Answer: B

The correct answer is between 20 and 30 breaths/minute. Note, this is inbetween a neonate and an adolescent's rates.

396. Answer: A

The correct answer is 1/5 to 1/10 that of an adolescent. As the baby grows, new terminal bronchioles and alveoli will form in the distal airways. Hmm..may explain why second hand smoke is so bad for babies!

397. Answer: C

The correct answer is carbon monoxide poisoning. All the workers were diagnosed as suffering from carbon monoxide poisoning. CO has been called the silent killer and has been the cause of approximately 5,000 deaths annually, with 2 to 5 times that requiring treatment. Even with treatment, the devastating sequelae that can accompany CO poisoning can be life changing. These include chorea, rigidity, dementia, myoclonus, impaired sensory function, seizures, and gait dysfunction. There can also be permanent cardiac damage due to the hypoxia involved in the poisoning process.

CO is an odorless, colorless and tasteless gas that results from incomplete combustion of fuels (i.e., coal, wood, gasoline). Once inhaled it binds quickly and tightly to the hemoglobin (Hgb), crowds out the oxygen and studies have shown CO can bind 200 times stronger than oxygen. Since the Hgb can no longer carry the oxygen the patient becomes hypoxemic and anoxic. Also the CO binds with myoglobin in the muscles and interferes with cellular metabolism causing metabolic acidosis.

Normal carboxyhemoglobin (HbCO) levels are 0% to 3% for non-smokers and 3% to 8% for smokers. A level of 10% to 20% causes headaches, nausea, vomiting and dyspnea. 30% to 40% causes severe headaches, syncope, and tachy-arrhythmias. Greater than 40% causes Cheyne-Stokes respiration or respiratory failure, seizures, unconsciousness, permanent brain damage, cardiac arrest and even death.

Because of the vagueness of the symptoms and their similarity to flu-like symptoms (N-V, dizziness, headache, etc.) CO poisoning is often misdiagnosed. Also, even if HbCO is present, it cannot be diagnosed with a simple pulse oximetry device because the displayed saturation level equals the sum of the oxyhemoglobin and carboxyhemoglobin.

So, if a patient comes to you and CO poisoning is suspected, what should you do? First and foremost, the patient needs high flow, high concentration O2, preferably a non-rebreather mask at 15 liters per minute, also a large bore IV. Prepare for blood draws (ABG, CBC, Lytes, CPK, Lactate, & Carboxyhemoglobin), a urine sample is also useful to rule out rhabdomyolysis (cardiac muscle breakdown secondary to the myoglobin damage from CO).

Other treatment modalities may include a CXR, cardiac monitoring and possibly Mannitol (1-2G/kg) to help decrease the cerebral edema accompanying the CO poisoning. Lastly, but probably the most effective treatment, is transfer of the patient to a hyperbaric oxygen unit (HBO), this is clearly indicated when the patient is very symptomatic and or the HbCO is 25% or greater.

398. Answer: A

The correct answer is Ciprofloxacin. The problem is that he is on theophylline and adding ciprofloxacin has caused his theophylline clearance to decrease, thus resulting in increased serum levels of theophylline. The result of increased theophylline levels in the toxic range usually begins with nausea and vomiting. The other antibiotics do not induce changes in theophylline clearance. Oh yeah, astringimycin is not a real antibiotic so don't worry about having to go learn a whole new class of antibiotics.

399. Answer: A

The answer is low rate, small tidal volume, high flows. When ventilating an asthmatic patient the idea of "permissive hypercapnia" is important to remember. Focus on getting the oxygen saturation up and don't worry as much about the pCO_2. Each of the factors (low rate, small tidal volume, high flows) addresses the need for a prolonged expiratory phase. High flow on the inspiration allows for less time devoted to inspiration and more time to expiration. So based on the idea of "permissive hypercapnia" it makes sense to have a lower rate and smaller tidal volume.

400. Answer: E

The answer is family history. It would be exceedingly unusual for a male patient with cystic fibrosis to have children. The rest of the findings are consistent with CF. Remember that this gene is encoded on Chromosome 7. It causes a defect in sodium and chloride transport channels in lungs particularly, but also other organs.

401. Answer: A

Of the answers listed, the one that would NOT be an indication of removing mechanical ventilation is having a PEEP of 10 cm H_2O. PEEP should be less than 5 cm H_2O before discontinuation of mechanical ventilation and extubation can be considered. Vital capacity should be greater than 10 to 15 ml/kg. Tidal volume of 4 to 5 ml/kg is acceptable for removal from the ventilator. FiO_2 should be less than 40% before discontinuation of mechanical ventilation. $P(A-a)O_2$ at an FiO_2 of 100% less than 350 mm Hg for successful weaning off the ventilator and extubation.

402. Answer: B

The correct answer is pulmonary sarcoidosis. This patient has classic findings of pulmonary sarcoidosis. Her chest radiograph shows a diffuse miliary pattern, which is suspicious for tuberculous or metastatic carcinoma.

Her biopsy shows two small, non-necrotizing granulomas.
The differential diagnosis includes mainly infectious granulomatous disease, hypersensitivity pneumonia, and sarcoidosis. Granulomas may also be seen with aspiration pneumonia, in chronic beryllium disease or exposure to titanium or aluminum dusts, as a response to certain drugs, and rarely with Wegener's granulomatosis, lymphocytic interstitial pneumonia or eosinophilic pneumonia.

Tuberculosis has been effectively ruled out at this point and bacterial pneumonia does not fit this clinical picture or any of the results. Asbestosis would cause parenchymal fibrosis and involves lower lobes. The bronchoscopy findings are inconsistent with asbestosis. Wegener's is on the differential, as mentioned above, but we have no evidence of renal disease and it is much rarer than Sarcoid in the African-American population.

403. Answer: C

This patient has had a pulmonary embolism. There is an increased risk of thromboembolic disease during pregnancy with possible contributing factors including:

Decreased vasomotor tone due to increased prostaglandins
Venous compression by the gravid uterus
Hypercoagulability due to increased levels of coagulation factors I, II, VIII, IX, and X.
Decreased plasma fibrinolytic activity.

This patient had her onset of pulmonary embolism approximately 1 week ago. Thrombolytic therapy is as effective if started in 6-14 days as compared to within 5 days of pulmonary embolism.

Her ECG is classic. The S1, Q3, T3 pattern is what is classically described but usually not seen. Echocardiogram is consistent with PE. With treatment and resolution her tricuspid regurgitation disappeared. Her right ventricle also returned to normal size as did her pulmonary artery systolic pressure. Because of her age you would also look for evidence of protein C or S deficiency.

404. Answer: A

The correct answer is to admit to the hospital, place chest tube and start intravenous ceftriaxone. He has an empyema by definition: he has organisms seen on gram stain! The organism is likely pneumococcus. Because he has an empyema you must place the chest tube as soon as possible; he will not get better without drainage of the pus. Intravenous antibiotics alone will not work. Waiting 24 hours or consulting a pulmonologist will not change the basic fact that he needs "draino"!!! If you chose to send this patient home you get 20 lashes with a wet noodle. Remember organisms on gram stain of pleural fluid = NEEDS CHEST TUBE. Finally, the choice to add gentamicin for synergy is not correct. It is only useful for synergy for *Staphylococcus*, group B *Streptococcus*, *Listeria*, and *Enterococcus* infections.

405. Answer: A

The answer is *Staphylococcus aureus*. She has had recent influenza and this is the classic setting where Staphylococcal pneumonia will occur. *Streptococcus pneumoniae* is still very common in these patients also. Influenza virus is known both to increase respiratory colonization by *S. aureus* and to impair ciliary function (and therefore clearance of staphylococci).

406. Answer: D

The correct answer is to continue current therapy. Clinically she is doing well; you are weaning her off the vent; her physical examination is stable; her laboratory is stable (NEVER BASE ANTIBIOTIC THERAPY on a MINOR BUMP IN WBC). The sputum results are not unusual for a patient in the Intensive Care Unit; they will frequently become colonized with gram-negative organisms—particularly *Pseudomonas*. Never change therapy based on just a tracheal aspirate..you must have some other change in exam or laboratory that is significant for you to consider treating the organism found on a tracheal aspirate.

407. Answer: A

The answer is *Francisella tularensis*. You need to put together the following: He is from Arkansas—if you see this State think: Blastomycosis, Histoplasmosis, Ehrlichiosis and Tularemia (a mnemonic for those of you mnemonically driven: BHET: Bill and Hilary Eat Toads in Arkansas). 2nd he is a hunter in Arkansas: say the 4 organisms again! 3rd he has a pneumonia that is unresponsive to ceftriaxone—think an unusual organism which could be any of our 4 choices (BHET). Finally, they tell you he is growing a gram-negative rod. Put Arkansas, pneumonia and gram-negative rod together and there is only one choice: Tularemia which is caused by *Francisella tularensis*.

408. Answer: A

Ok. If you didn't get the right answer here get on the floor and give me 50 pushups. If you see the words pneumonia and San Joaquin Valley go for Coccidioidomycosis (by the way do you know how difficult it is to spell and type Coccidioidomycosis?? Try it. The spell checker at MedStudy is tired just from me using this dang word so many times in this one question.). Now read the question though because occasionally -very occasionally- they will throw in a simple Pneumococcal pneumonia on someone who lives in a weird part (Oops..sorry if you are from the San Joaquin Valley. I don't mean that you are "weird"—you know what I mean) of the country just to be sure you know that common things are common and rare things are rare. BUT, they will make it very clear they have something mundane like pneumococcal pneumonia: fever, a shaking chill, rusty sputum, etc....

409. Answer: C

The correct answer is *Chlamydia pneumoniae*. With the history of prior sore throat and now a febrile illness with documented pneumonia by chest x-ray; *Chlamydia pneumoniae* is the most likely. The stupid parrot is a red herring here as she had no signs of *C. psittaci* infection—look for a pneumonia with an extensive interstitial pattern that appears to be much worse than the physical exam would indicate. *C. trachomatis* remember, causes genitourinary disease. *Staphylococcal aureus* would be seen after an influenza-like illness or if she were immunocompromised and she would be much sicker. Don't be thrown by the positive throat culture for this organism---it can be found frequently in asymptomatic people. *H. influenzae* should not cause pneumonia in her age group.

410. Answer: B

The answer is azithromycin. She could have *Streptococcus pneumoniae, Mycoplasma pneumoniae, or Chlamydia pneumoniae*. Azithromycin and gatifloxacin are the only agents listed that are effective against all 3 organisms. The problem is that she is 17—note the ABP will follow the FDA rules. You cannot give a quinolone to a child under the age of 18 except in special circumstances (anthrax, Cystic Fibrosis patients, etc.). The Beta-lactam antibiotics listed are great for pneumococcus but won't get the atypicals. In an adolescent with uncomplicated pneumonia, look for a macrolide or doxycycline as an acceptable choice.

411. Answer: D

The answer is to start INH 300mg daily for 9 months. He is a recent converter. He has had a 10 mm increase in 1 year's time. By definition, he should receive prophylaxis. His CXR is normal and he has no signs or symptoms of tuberculosis, therefore, he does not need to be treated for active tuberculosis. 12 months of INH is no longer recommended for anyone, including HIV-infected patients! It is not reasonable to repeat the PPD in 2 weeks; he has a positive result. It will not change with repeated testing.

412. Answer: A

The answer is a PPD containing 5 TU of tuberculin without controls. The use of "control" testing is no longer recommended by the American Thoracic Society or the CDC for any patient routinely. Therefore, the use of controls should be discouraged. Even though she is severely immunocompromised, a standard PPD is still appropriate. NEVER EVER pick the 250 TU on a test. There is no reason to use it so you can effectively mark out those answers when you see them listed on a test! The 2 step (or boosted) PPD has no place in routine practice; it is generally reserved for people who are repeatedly tested, such as health care workers.

413. Answer: A

The person who should NOT receive prophylaxis therapy is the patient with the PPD reading at 72 hours of 7 mm who is immunocompromised with leukemia on 5mg/day of prednisone. According to the guidelines, the cut off is 10mm for this patient. All of the other patients require treatment; generally you would use INH for 9 months in each of these other patients. If this patient had been on 15 mg or more of daily prednisone then they would have met the criteria for therapy.

414. Answer: E

The answer is none needed unless clinical symptoms/problems develop. He is a healthy person without evidence of liver disorder. If, during the initial evaluation, he had evidence to suggest a liver disorder, then he should have baseline serum aspartate aminotransferase (AST) or serum alanine aminotransferase (ALT) and bilirubin drawn. Baseline testing is also indicated for patients with HIV infection, pregnant women, and women in the immediate postpartum period (within 3 months of delivery), persons with a history of chronic liver disease (hepatitis B or C, alcoholic hepatitis, or cirrhosis), persons who use alcohol regularly, and persons at risk for chronic liver disease. Baseline testing is NO LONGER routinely indicated in older persons (>35y/o). But, for patients with chronic conditions on medications that could cause problems, testing may be warranted. Guidelines do not say how often to do laboratory testing but probably q monthly is a good idea in those patients who require baseline screening.

Now clinical monitoring is indicated! This includes educating patients about signs and symptoms that might indicate a problem with the medication. These include any of the following: unexplained anorexia, nausea, vomiting, dark urine, icterus, rash, persistent paresthesias of the hand and feet, persistent fatigue, weakness or fever lasting 3 or more days, abdominal tenderness (especially right upper quadrant discomfort), easy bruising or bleeding, and arthralgia. Clinical monitoring begins at the first visit and should be done monthly.

415. Answer: C

The answer is ethambutol toxicity. Ethambutol is generally not hepatotoxic but will cause problems with visual acuity, particularly color perceptions. The other agents are not associated with this problem.

416. Answer: D

The answer is *Coxiella burnetii*. For this case, the fact that he worked with animal placentas should make you think about *Coxiella burnetii*—remember, if you see some type of animal "placenta" or birthing event, then consider *Coxiella burnetii*—recent literature has had outbreaks with CATS—so be suspicious if Tabby is around delivering kittens and people are getting pneumonia. The other clue that this might be *Coxiella* is the marked hepatosplenomegaly. This is one of those "pneumonia with splenomegaly" organisms.

417. Answer: E

The correct answer is systemic corticosteroids. The key here is that she has Allergic Bronchopulmonary Aspergillosis (ABPA). The treatment for this is steroids and not anti-fungal agents. If you see something fungal that is branching, it is likely aspergillus especially if there is "right-angle" or 90 degree branching.

418. Answer: E

The answer is no further workup is needed. Calcified nodules are benign. And in this patient, being that he is from Mississippi; histoplasmosis is a likely etiology. They do not require further workup. If he had a "popcorn" calcified pattern then you would schedule followup CXR over a period of 2 years to be sure it didn't get bigger; as this is likely a hamartoma. Solitary nodules WITHOUT calcifications are also watched for 2 years in low-risk patients (on the TEST)—in the real world we all know we work these things up and the answer is: Benign 99% of the time).

419. Answer: B

The correct answer is alveolar hypoventilation alone. The differential diagnosis of arterial hypoxemia includes all of the above plus decreased diffusion and high altitude (low FiO2). While this patient is at risk for aspiration pneumonia, pulmonary edema and other underlying pulmonary pathology, a quick calculation of the A-a gradient on room air reveals a normal A-a gradient. (150- (50+ 72/0.8) = A-a gradient of 10. The A-a gradient is increased in all causes of hypoxemia except hypoventilation and high altitude. We were not given any information that this patient was found on the summit of a mountain in Aspen, therefore, alveolar hypoventilation due to the presumed narcotic injection is the physiological mechanism for hypoxemia in this patient.

420. Answer: A

The correct answer is bronchoprovocation (Methacholine challenge test). With a normal cardiovascular and pulmonary exam, the most likely cause of the episodic dyspnea in this patient under 40 years of age is asthma. As asthma is episodic and reversible airway obstruction, spirometry performed while the patient is asymptomatic may well be normal. The best test to prove asthma is the methacholine bronchoprovocation test which will reveal hyper-reactive airways – the hallmark of asthma. If the patient had rales on the exam and was older, the possibility of an interstitial lung disease would have to be entertained and an HRCT of the chest would be indicated. Remember, 10% of patients with interstitial lung disease will have a normal chest x-ray at the time of presentation. If the patient gave a history of chest pain or syncope with exertion and physical exam revealed a right parasternal heave and an accentuated P2 then the diagnosis of pulmonary hypertension by echocardiography would be warranted. If an upper airway obstruction was suggested by the history or the patient was found to have stridor, a Flow-Volume Loop would be a good screening test for upper airway obstruction. A normal ABG with a normal A-a gradient would make a diffusing capacity limitation unlikely.

421. Answer: C

The correct answer is inhaled corticosteroid, twice daily plus B-2 agonist as needed. This patient has asthma which would be characterized as Moderate-Persistent by the National Asthma Education and Prevention Program Guidelines. As such, she should be on daily medication with an inhaled corticosteroid and a short acting inhaled B-2 agonist as needed for symptoms. The emphasis on utilizing anti-inflammatory therapies (inhaled corticosteroids) was a major focus on the NAEPP guidelines for any asthma patient characterized as mild-persistent or greater. This was to overcome the over-reliance on symptomatic relief with B-2 agonist inhalers and the rising number of asthma deaths (most clutching their B-agonist inhalers and on no steroids!). A B-2 agonist inhaler must be available for symptomatic relief with the understanding that more frequent use of the B-agonist inhaler indicates a need for stepped-up anti-inflammatory therapy (higher dose inhaled sterids, PO prednisone). Long acting B-agonist inhalers may be helpful but cannot be used for immediate relief of symptoms in an acute exacerbation. This means your patient would need three inhalers – an inhaled corticosteroid as well as both long acting and short acting B-2 agonist inhalers. Sustained release theophylline may help with nocturnal symptoms but has no anti-inflammatory action. Inhaled cromolyn alone can take weeks to start working and is best used in atopic asthma in children.

422. Answer: D

The correct answer is delayed (type IV, cell mediated) skin test reaction to *A. fumigatus.* All of the above are considered minor or major criteria for the diagnosis of ABPA except that there is no type IV cell-mediated skin reaction. There are Type I and Type III (erythema and induration) skin test reactions. ABPA should be a consideration in any asthmatic who clinically worsens with repeated attacks despite adherence to therapy.

423. Answer: B

The correct answer is echocardiogram. Look for the young woman with exertional dyspnea, chest pain and has physical exam findings consistent with right heart strain. The next step in the workup is an echocardiogram to document the existence of pulmonary hypertension and exclude significant mitral stenosis. After echocardiographic documentation of pulmonary hypertension, the workup would proceed in the absence of any discernible parenchymal lung disease on V/Q scan to look for thromboembolic disease. A pulmonary angiogram would be helpful in evaluating any perfusion defects seen on V/Q. The role of right heart catheterization is further down the road when you are considering vasodilator therapy in the patient with primary pulmonary hypertension.

424. Answer: E

The correct answer is no testing – observe the patient. You are going to get a question on histo or blastomycosis. I like this question as it keeps with the ABP's theme of doing nothing!
This patient has acute histoplasmosis from the neighborhood barn cleaning party. The neighborhood outbreak is not uncommon when there is land cleared or bulldozed.
The key is that histoplasmosis is usually a self-limited disease for which we do not consider treatment unless there is evidence for progression to more disseminated disease. Accurate diagnosis relies on the history of exposure. Histoplasmin skin tests are useless as many people will test positive after exposure without having disease. Cultures are not very sensitive and may take weeks to grow. A positive culture from sputum or tissue is diagnostic however. Serologic testing is not very sensitive and does not provide a timely diagnosis.

425. Answer: A

The correct answer is fixed split second sound. Most children with an ASD are asymptomatic although large defects can cause fatigue and rarely CHF. Clinical findings of an ASD consist of pulmonary ejection systolic murmur best heard at left upper sternal border, widely fixed split S2 (due to delayed closure of the pulmonic valve), and early to mid-diastolic rumble at the lower left sternal border (due to increased flow across tricuspid valve).

426. Answer: D

The correct answer is start prostaglandin E1 following echocardiography diagnosis. Cardiac cyanosis results from a fixed right-to-left shunt. The hyperoxia test was performed which differentiates between cardiac and other causes (pulmonary or metabolic). Failure of the arterial PO2 to increase to 100 to 150 mmHg after 100% O2 is administered for 10 minutes is usually indicative of cardiac origin of cyanosis. Although chest x-ray and EKG should be done at some point, immediate evaluation includes echocardiography followed by administration of prostaglandin E1 (if congenital cardiac disease identified) to keep the ductus arteriosus patent.

427. Answer: D

The answer is propranolol. Prolonged QT interval (heart rate-corrected QT interval > 0.45 sec) is caused by delayed ventricular repolarization. Usually these children present with a syncopal episode caused by exercise, fright, or a sudden startle. These patients are predisposed to life-threatening arrhythmias such as ventricular tachycardia and fibrillation. This patient definitely needs treatment to prevent these arrhythmias. Treatment with a beta-blocker (propranolol) is necessary to blunt the heart rate response to exercise. Both amiodarone and bretylium prolong repolarization. Ablation is used for accessory pathways in SVT.

428. Answer: C

The correct answer is transposition of the great vessels. Cyanosis is usually noted in the first day of life and progresses rapidly as the ductus arteriosus closes. Remember with this the aorta comes off the right ventricle and the pulmonary artery from the left. Tetralogy of Fallot is the more common but it won't show up till later in childhood. A trick question—how evil of me. But the Boards want you to think on the exam also. Think about the anatomy—a baby is born with transposition—he/she will be cyanotic very quickly. With Tetralogy the cyanosis won't occur for a while until the right ventricular outflow obstruction is progressive - usually not for the first few months of life. Later the kids get what is known as "tet" spells. These spells are hypoxic events and the child becomes restless and agitated and may cry inconsolably. Frequently, children learn early on to "squat" and that helps increase systemic venous return resulting in more blood being made available to the pulmonary artery and increases systemic resistance, driving more venous blood into the lungs. Total anomalous pulmonary venous return is when there is a failure of incorporation of the common pulmonary vein into the posterior wall of the left atrium; this will cause severe cyanosis in the newborn period but is rarer than transposition. Tricuspid atresia will not usually cause cyanosis till around a year of age due to the presence of a VSD with this abnormality. VSD will not cause a cyanotic disease usually.

429. Answer: A

The correct answer is large VSD, right ventricular outflow tract obstruction, overriding aorta, RVH. This is just a simple memorization thing. It has appeared on past tests so just memorize it. A pneumonic that helps me but may not you is: "VROARV"; where V stands for VSD, RO stands for right ventricular outflow obstruction, OA for overriding aorta, and RV for RVH. Like I said it may or may not help you—my brain is weird sometimes how it works.

430. Answer: C

The correct answer is to do a Holter study. She likely is having an arrhythmia (such as SVT) from her caffeine intake. The best test would be to monitor on a Holter and then see what arrhythmia is occurring. The other tests are not indicated at this time.

431. Answer: E

The correct answer is hypertrophic cardiomyopathy. All of the other choices do not require prophylaxis. You would think that having a pacer with electrodes going directly into the heart would, but there is no increased risk. The systolic click alone does not warrant prophylaxis either; a murmur also is required. Ok, you ask about the stupid coronary artery surgery and implanted defibrillator? These are adult things right?? Well, consider the kid with Kawasaki who had coronary artery surgery or the post-op funny looking kid with the congenital heart disease who keeps going into v-fib and needs the defibrillator—it can happen!

432. Answer: B

The correct answer is initial placement of orthodontic bands. Evidently this is enough manipulation of the gums to produce enough trauma where prophylaxis is indicated. All of the other items listed do not require prophylaxis. It is comforting to know that every time people go in for their orthodontic "adjustment" that prophylaxis is not indicated.

433. Answer: B

The correct answer is hypertrophic obstructive cardiomyopathy (HOCM or IHSS). The combination of...

- A. "spike and dome" carotid pulse contour
- B. similar apex cardiogram
- C. holosystolic murmur
- D. murmur augmentation by standing and ...
- E. murmur augmentation by Valsalva strain
- F. the Brockenbrough phenomenon
- G. sudden death (resuscitated)

Makes the diagnosis of hypertrophic (obstructive) cardiomyopathy inescapable here. The pure form of this disease is now known to be an autosomal dominant transmission, this explaining the importance of investigation of other members of the kindred, particularly in the type of scenario described. This entity is one of the several diagnoses that is customarily first considered when there is an acute event in an elite athlete, other entities worth consideration in this regard being WPW, Marfan physiology, anomalous coronary disease and long QT_c syndrome.

Appropriate associations with the other entities mentioned might include:

- A. myxomatous mitral valve prolapse [MVP] - mid-systolic click
- B. ostium secundum atrial septal defect [ASD] - fixed splitting of S_{II}
- C. ostium primum atrioventricular septal defect [AVSD] - RBBB / LAHB
- D. acquired (muscular) ventricular septal defect [VSD] - myocardial infarction
- E. Wolff-Parkinson-White syndrome [WPW] - delta waves
- F. congenital long QT syndrome (Romano-Ward) - QT_c > 0.43-0.44

434. Answer: A

The correct answer is tricuspid regurgitation. The patients of this nature are so familiar in some geographic settings that the diagnosis is nearly routine. The characteristic features of tricuspid regurgitation accompanied by septic pulmonary emboli and evidence of parenteral drug usage predict that *Staphylococcus aureus* will be isolated as the causative agent in the majority of cases. Some of these patients have even had their tricuspid valves removed rather than attempting to implant a prosthetic device in a patient who could return to bacteremia-associated behaviors (via relapse). This is something that can be done if the patient has no additional heart disease. An alternative to this approach might include a plastic repair of the native valve, a so-called "vegetectomy."

435. Answer: B

The correct answer is they must be aware of the risk of sudden death. Unfortunately, this is very much the truth, and indeed most boys with classical Duchenne's muscular dystrophy will not live past 20 years. It is precisely for this reason that there are fundamentally no girls with the disease, despite the predictions of the Punnett Square; there are (literally) no fathers! Whereas the cause of death in many Duchenne boys will be the relentless chronic progression of cardiopulmonary disease, there is an important component of sudden death relating to the arrhythmias and conduction system disease accompanying their characteristic cardiomyopathy. The EKG has been a topic of extraordinary interest in these patients in that they invariably display a completely unique "pseudo-infarction" pattern of posterolateral changes representing a genetically determined focal myocardial scar. In addition, they display so-called "high-frequency notches" [HFN] and tend to have a small number of HFN in the early stages of the disease; with increasing severity of the disease they develop a larger number, and in the terminal stage they again exhibit relatively few notches. It is felt that significant increases or decreases in the count of HFN on QRS complexes can be useful indicators for estimating the extent and severity of cardiac involvement in progressive muscular dystrophy.

436. Answer: C

The correct answer is ostium secundum atrial septal defect (ASD). Again, from a test-taker's point of view, the noting of fixed splitting of the second heart sound means that only one answer is possible on a test. In "real-life," there are occasional patients with ventricular septal defect who have this finding, but that would never be the point on an examination of this quality. The flow murmur is typical and represents the shunt volume in the pulmonary artery. In fact, there may be a murmur resulting from the flow across the septal defect itself, but this is, in fact, a diastolic murmur, and is seldom heard clinically.

This phenomenon is also largely exhalation-dependent and is therefore, nonetheless, exactly what explains the fixed splitting: Whereas <u>inspiration</u> volume loads the right ventricle in the usual fashion (via acceleration of caval flow), <u>expiration</u> volume loads the right ventricle again (via the increase in shunt volume across the septal defect itself in exhalation), thereby resulting in a balance of loading phenomena affecting the right heart (and effectively "holding" P_2 away from A_2).

437. Answer: E

The answer is no abnormalities. There has been heightened awareness of sudden death of young people partaking in strenuous exercise after several highly publicized episodes. The largest series of autopsies in these individuals have shown no abnormalities in the majority of patients. Death was presumably due to a ventricular arrhythmia from an unrecognized source, possibly a subclinical cardiomyopathy or an unknown genetic disorder.
If any abnormality is found on autopsy, hypertrophic cardiomyopathy is the commonest, followed by anomalous origin of the coronary arteries.

438. Answer: D

The correct answer is a sound heard with the diaphragm at the apex shortly after S2. This actress was portraying someone with rheumatic mitral stenosis. There would likely be an opening snap heard at the apex after S2. The opening snap is a high-pitched sound, and thus heard better with the diaphragm. S1 is typically loud in mitral stenosis. Aortic regurgitation would produce a decrescendo blowing murmur at the left lower sternal border with the patient sitting forward. Mitral valve prolapse would present with the click and murmur. A sound heard with the bell at the apex after S2 would be an S3, which patients with mitral stenosis are very unlikely to have, since the left ventricle is not filled rapidly.

439. Answer: A

The correct answer is open airway and check breathing. Always remember your ABCs. Start with airway, breathing, then circulation. Although this child will probably need intubation, you must first assess the airway and breathing.

440. Answer: D

The correct answer is establish vascular access to administer adenosine. This patient has supraventricular tachycardia (SVT) with adequate perfusion that allows a trial of vagal maneuvers while IV access is established to administer adenosine. Adenosine temporarily blocks conduction through the AV node for about 10 seconds. SVT is most commonly caused by a reentry mechanism involving the AV conduction system or accessory pathway. Had the patient been unstable, immediate cardioversion would have been required.

441. Answer: B

The correct answer is congestive heart failure. Remember these patients have a RIGHT to LEFT shunt. They are likely to get cyanosis, hypoxemia and resulting poor growth. They do not have increased pulmonary blood flow nor left ventricular obstruction. The 'tet' spells result from an acute increase in right to left shunting and can be triggered by a reduction in systemic arterial resistance or by an increase in right ventricular outflow obstruction. Brain abscesses are a well-known complication of cyanotic congenital heart disease.

442. Answer: B

The correct answer is supraventricular tachycardia without underlying congenital heart disease. Heart rates over 200 are rarely sinus tachycardia—so mark that one off. The QRS complexes are described as normal—that should eliminate ventricular fibrillation and we will assume that they are not "wide-complex" so ventricular tachycardia is also not likely—especially with this heart rate. Most infants who present with SVT (which this child is at the peak age and is usually associated with a respiratory infection), do not have associated structural heart abnormalities.

443. Answer: A

The correct answer is *viridans Streptococci*, Enterococcus, and *Staphylococcus aureus*. Nearly ½ are due to the group viridans Streptococci, which includes *S. mitior* and *S. sanguis*.

444. Answer: E

The correct answer is total anomalous pulmonary venous return with obstruction of the veins. Ok, lets review: remember, the pulmonary veins drain to the right atrium instead of the left atrium. Then there is mixing with the systemic venous return in the right atrium. Next, some of the oxygenated pulmonary venous blood shunts across the foramen ovale, which provides a right-to-left shunt of partially oxygenated blood into the systemic circulation. In some cases—the pulmonary venous return is not directly into the right atrium, but instead takes a crazy course—like going below the diaphragm before reaching the right atrium. In this case, venous obstruction is likely. Although the heart may be considerably enlarged in those without venous obstruction, in those <u>with</u> venous obstruction it is usually normal or only minimally dilated.

445. Answer: B

The correct answer is transposition of the great vessels. Let's review: In transposition, the aorta comes off of the right ventricle and the pulmonary artery comes off of the left ventricle. This causes 2 separate circulations—which is incompatible with life—unless there somehow is mixing or shunting of blood—like an ASD or VSD or a patent ductus arteriosus. An artificial ASD can be made by using a balloon and passing it through the foramen ovale. You then inflate the balloon and yank it—causing a communication between the left and the right atriums. It can be useful also for tricuspid or pulmonary atresia—but not for any of the other conditions listed.

446. Answer: D

The correct answer is Eisenmenger's syndrome. This occurs as a progressive increase in pulmonary vascular resistance, which can lead to a RIGHT-TO-LEFT shunt. In this situation, pulmonary vascular disease is irreversible and surgical closure of the defect is not helpful.

447. Answer: A

The correct answer is atrial septal defect. The ECG indicates right ventricular hypertrophy and all of the other findings are consistent with an ASD. Coarctation of the aorta and VSD would give you Left ventricular hypertrophy.

448. Answer: A

The correct answer is an ECG in a 2-month-old infant. An Rs pattern over the right precordium of an infant or child less than 2 is a reflection of the normal right ventricular predominance for that age.

449. Answer: C

The correct answer is both a 12 year-old and a 2 month old child's ECG. The T waves are inverted in V_3R through V_3 in most infants and can remain inverted in V_3R to V_1 up to about age 15 years.

450. Answer: D

The correct answer is it is never normal except in the first few days of life.

451. Answer: E

The correct answer is this is never normal. In an infant or child, an inverted P wave in Lead I can indicate dextrocardia!

452. Answer: B

The correct answer is transposition of the great vessels with a VSD. In transposition of the great vessels the output of the right ventricle enters the aorta and returns to the right atrium. The output of the left ventricle flows to the lungs and from there to the left atrium. These two independent circulations are incompatible with life unless there is mixing between the two circulations. Cyanosis occurs from the right-to-left component of the mixing and congestive heart failure occurs due to left ventricular output flowing to the lungs.

A large VSD by itself would just produce congestive heart failure due to left-to-right shunting and markedly increased pulmonary blood flow.

Tetralogy of Fallot is characterized by a right to left shunt at the ventricular level. This results in persistent cyanosis. Pulmonary blood flow however is decreased and there is no obstruction to left ventricular outflow therefore, no CHF is evident.

ASD causes a left-to-right shunt and therefore no cyanosis. The pressure gradient is small so CHF is very unlikely.

Double aortic arch is a congenital malformation that results in a "vascular ring" which encircles the trachea. Symptoms are due to compression of the trachea and include primarily inspiratory stridor –but it does not produce cyanosis nor CHF.

453. Answer: D

The correct answer is large VSD in a 6-month-old. A large VSD by itself would just produce congestive heart failure due to left-to-right shunting and markedly increased pulmonary blood flow.

In transposition of the great vessels, the output of the right ventricle enters the aorta and returns to the right atrium. The output of the left ventricle flows to the lungs and from there to the left atrium. These two independent circulations are incompatible with life unless there is mixing between the two circulations. Cyanosis occurs from the right-to-left component of the mixing and congestive heart failure occurs due to left ventricular output flowing to the lungs.

Tetralogy of Fallot is characterized by a right to left shunt at the ventricular level. This results in persistent cyanosis. Pulmonary blood flow however is decreased and there is no obstruction to left ventricular outflow, therefore, no CHF is evident.

ASD causes a left-to-right shunt and therefore no cyanosis. The pressure gradient is small so CHF is very unlikely.

Double aortic arch is a congenital malformation that results in a "vascular ring" which encircles the trachea. Symptoms are due to compression of the trachea and include primarily inspiratory stridor –but it does not produce cyanosis or CHF.

454. Answer: A

The correct answer is congestive heart failure is possible. In bacterial endocarditis, CHF is usually due to valvular destruction and resultant insufficiency while in acute rheumatic fever it is usually due to myocarditis. Subcutaneous nodules and erythema marginatum are seen in acute rheumatic fever. Petechiae are only associated with endocarditis (embolic phenomenon). Neither will have a macrocytic, hypochromic anemia. Both can have a mild anemia but it is usually normocytic, normochromic.

455. Answer: A

The correct answer is Pompe's disease. CHF commonly occurs within the first 2 years with Pompe's disease. In Marfan's syndrome, cardiac symptoms rarely develop before the age of 5. In Friedreich's ataxia, symptoms are rare in infancy and cardiac failure at any age is uncommon—arrhythmias and electrocardiographic abnormalities are more common.

456. Answer: D

The correct answer is a diastolic murmur. A diastolic murmur is not a common finding in Tetralogy of Fallot. Many of the features are due to a right-to-left shunt—clubbing, cyanosis and polycythemia. Episodes that suddenly will increase the right-to-left shunt result in "tet" spells and anoxia. The murmur and thrill are due to the VSD. Children with tetralogy will squat with physical exertion or afterwards to help increase systemic vascular resistance and decrease the magnitude of the right-to-left shunt.

457. Answer: E

The correct answer is right ventricular hypertrophy. Aortic pressure is greatly more than pulmonary pressure, right? Therefore, a patent ductus arteriosus will give you a continuous left-to-right shunt and therefore a continuous murmur. The increased left ventricular output with run-off from the aorta through the ductus produces the widened pulse pressure and a bounding pulse. The increased flow to the lungs and back to the left ventricle causes hypertrophy of the left ventricle rather than the right ventricle.

458. Answer: B

The correct "incorrect" answer is spontaneous closure of the ductus arteriosus in infancy will produce improvement in symptoms. This is not true—it will produce worsening of symptoms. Why? Let's review. Coarctation always occurs near the insertion of the ductus arteriosus. In most cases, the "shelf" of narrowing is directly opposite the orifice of the ductus. This way, aortic blood flow can bypass the coarctation by flowing through the orifice or proximal portion of the ductus and then around the protruding aortic "shelf". Now, when the ductus closes spontaneously—this bypass doesn't exist anymore and obstruction becomes more severe. CHF can develop early (3-6 months) or be delayed until adulthood. All of the other items listed are true.

459. Answer: E

The correct answer is it usually heals without deformity. The arthritis of acute rheumatic fever is a painful, acute migratory polyarthritis. Usually the large joints are involved. Fever and arthritis usually occur at the same time.

460. Answer: D

The correct answer is fine tremor is noted. This is usually not seen with chorea. Seizures are also not seen with chorea either. Everything else listed is associated or seen with chorea. (I must have had chorea as a child based on my handwriting grades in elementary school—hmm..better yet, I must still have chorea!).

461. Answer: C

The correct answer is 95/60. It pretty much stays in this range until 6 years of age. After that it gradually increases until the age of 12 when it generally is about 120/70.

462. Answer: D

The correct answer is a shorter PR interval and a shorter RR interval. Remember that the heart rate of an infant is considerably faster than that of an adolescent. This increased rate is associated with a shorter PR interval and a shorter RR interval.

463. Answer: A

The correct answer is transposition of the great vessels with a ventricular septal defect (VSD). If the patient did not have a VSD this patient would have presented in the immediate newborn period due to having an independent parallel circulation and the life of the baby would have been dependent on establishing some mixing of the two circulations. Because this patient has a VSD, the patient is asymptomatic until there is a drop in pulmonary resistance through natural maturation. Once this occurs, the blood will shunt from right to left through the ventricular defect. Because the left ventricle relates to the pulmonary circulation, it will have lower pressure thus leading to the right to left shunting. This increased flow will lead to the increased pulmonary marking demonstrated on this chest x-ray. Since the right ventricle relates to the systemic system, right ventricular hypertrophy develops. The mediastinum is narrow because the great vessels do not completely change position but relate in an anterior-posterior direction. Patients with truncus arteriosus are cyanotic at birth. Patients with total anomalous pulmonary venous return will have a small heart on chest x-ray. Tricuspid atresia patients will also be cyanotic but will have a left axis deviation with left ventricular hypertrophy on EKG. The patient with tetralogy of Fallot will have decreased vascular markings and a boot shaped heart.

464. Answer: A

The correct answer is atrial septal defect. The patient with an atrial septal defect has a burden placed on the right side of the heart resulting in an increased blood volume from the left atrium to the right atrium. This increased blood flow results in an increase in the right atrium, right ventricle, and pulmonary artery. The fixed overload on the right ventricle results in a prolonged ejection time of the chamber and consequently delaying of the closure of the pulmonary valve. This results in a wide split of the second heart sound. The classic murmur with a ventricular septal defect is a holosystolic murmur located at the fourth intercostal space to the left of the sternum with a normal second heart sound. The murmur of pulmonary stenosis will be less harsh than an atrial septal defect and there should be no splitting of the second heart sound. A patient with an innocent murmur will have a normal second heart sound and the murmur will vary considerably with changes in position and exercise. The murmur of a patent ductus arteriosus is a continuous murmur usually present in the first months of life.

465. Answer: C

The correct answer is Eisenmenger's complex. Eisenmenger's complex is a clinical situation when a patient has a left to right shunt (e.g., ventricular septal defect) that goes unrepaired long enough that the patient develops an increase in the pulmonary vascular resistance and develops pulmonary hypertension. Once this occurs the shunt changes from left to right to right to left. In such a situation the chest x-ray would demonstrate changes consistent with an enlarged right atrium, right ventricle, and pulmonary artery and the EKG would demonstrate right ventricular hypertrophy. Tricuspid atresia and total anomalous pulmonary venous return would have been present since birth. The chest x-ray of tetralogy of Fallot would have demonstrated a decrease in pulmonary vascular markings and most individuals with an atrial septal defect are asymptomatic.

466. Answer: E

The correct answer is coarctation of the aorta. This lesion is not usually confused with any others. This patient would have a post ductal coarctation and if a blood pressure had been taken in his legs it would have been diminished. The classic murmur which is audible on the posterior aspect of the chest and the rib notching on chest x-ray eliminate the other choices. Rib notching does not usually occur prior to 8 years of age and is a function of physical erosion of the under surface of the ribs due to the increased intercostal circulation. A bruit can be audible due to the collateral flow through the dilated intercostal arteries in the posterior aspect of the chest and the dilated mammary arteries in the anterior aspect of the chest.

467. Answer: B

The correct answer is a patent ductus arteriosus (PDA). The classic continuous murmur should make one think of a PDA. A venous hum is an innocent phenomenon that relates to the venous return. The venous hum will usually disappear when the patient is lying down whereas the murmur of the PDA will remain or increase when lying down. The murmur associated with pulmonary artery stenosis is usually best heard under the clavicles. The murmur of an atrial septal defect is an ejection murmur and the ventricular septal defect will have a holosystolic murmur heard throughout the chest.

468. Answer: B

The correct answer is tetralogy of Fallot. Tetralogy of Fallot is comprised of right ventricular hypertrophy, pulmonary stenosis, ventricular septal defect, and an overriding aorta. This baby was having "tet spells" which are cyanotic episodes due to shunting of blood right to left across the ventricular septal defect. Severe pulmonary stenosis would present with constant cyanosis and the baby is not old enough to develop Eisenmenger's complex. The chest x-ray and EKG should be normal in patients with a simple ventricular septal defect. Tricuspid atresia can be confused with tetralogy of Fallot early in infancy but should have left ventricular hypertrophy on EKG.

469. Answer: A

The correct answer is tricuspid atresia. Any of the other lesions should be strongly considered but the presence of left ventricular hypertrophy on the EKG virtually eliminates all of the other lesions from consideration.

470. Answer: B

The correct answer is total anomalous pulmonary venous return (TAPVR). The patient with total anomalous pulmonary venous return without obstruction is usually symptomatic as an infant whereas the infant with TAPVR with obstruction is usually symptomatic at birth. The diagnosis of TAPVR should be suspected in a patient with relatively poor growth and developmental delay. A systolic ejection murmur high along the left chest, a mild diastolic murmur low along the left side of the chest, and a widely split second heart sound are commonly demonstrated in such patients. A chest x-ray demonstrating right atrial and right ventricular enlargement with increased vascular markings is usually evident. The presence of the "Snowman" configuration on chest x-ray is the classic finding. Patients with an atrial septal defect will have a similar clinical presentation but should not have an enlarged mediastinum. Patients with a ventricular septal defect have a classic murmur (3-4/6 holosystolic murmur) along the left sternal border. Truncus arteriosus might be the most confusing to differentiate from TAPVR but these patients will usually have a single second heart sound. Patients with an atrioventricular canal will usually have left axis deviation and biventricular hypertrophy on EKG.

471. Answer: B

The correct answer is atrioventricular canal. This baby has features consistent with trisomy 21. An atrioventricular canal is the most common congenital cardiac lesion found in patients with trisomy 21. Cardiac signs and symptoms are often lacking early in life. Patients may have any type of murmur or none at all. A chest x-ray will usually demonstrate and enlarged heart with increased vascular markings. An EKG with an abnormal leftward axis and biventricular hypertrophy can also be demonstrated.

472. Answer: E

The correct answer is pulmonary valve stenosis. The patient described has Noonan syndrome. Noonan syndrome have the phenotypic features seen in Turner syndrome but have normal karyotypes. The cardiac defect that is most commonly demonstrated in Noonan syndrome is pulmonary valvular stenosis but hypertrophic cardiomyopathy and atrial septal defects can also be demonstrated. The murmur described above is that of severe pulmonary valvular stenosis.

473. Answer: D

The correct answer is non-stenotic bicuspid aortic valve. The patient described has Turner syndrome. This syndrome is found in girls with the same phenotypic features including short stature, webbed neck, and cubitus valgus. These girls usually only have "streak ovaries" present. One-third to one-half of patients with Turner syndrome have a non-stenotic bicuspid aortic valve. In later life, bicuspid aortic valve disease can progress to dilatation of the aortic root. Less frequent lesions include coarctation of the aorta (20%), aortic stenosis, and mitral valve prolapse.

474. Answer: A

The correct answer is supravalvular aortic stenosis. Supravalvular aortic stenosis is an uncommon form of left ventricular obstruction and may be sporadic, familial or associated with William's syndrome. The patient described above has William's syndrome. William's syndrome included elfin facies, mental retardation, and idiopathic hypercalcemia of infancy.

475. Answer: A

The correct answer is 17-alpha-hydroxyprogesterone (17OHP) and electrolytes. CAH is a group of genetic disorders of adrenal steroid biosynthesis. There are varying degrees of the disease depending on the defects of the genes. Disorders of 21-hydroxylase (21-OH) deficiency account for approximately 95% of patients with CAH. The pathway for adrenal steroid hormone synthesis is complex, but since 21-OH deficiency accounts for most cases of CAH, it is most important to know that step. All steroid synthesis starts with cholesterol and goes through a series of conversions to form aldosterone, cortisol, testosterone and estradiol.

In the mineralocorticoid pathway, the inability to convert progesterone to 11-deoxycorticosterone (DOC) due to 21-OH deficiency results in aldosterone deficiency. Therefore the kidney cannot retain sodium normally and serum sodium concentration can fall to the low 100s. The kidney also inappropriately retains K+ and H+ resulting in hyperkalemia, acidosis, hypotension, shock, cardiovascular collapse and death.

In the glucocorticoid pathway, the inability to convert 17OH progesterone to 11-deoxycortisol due to 21-OH deficiency results in cortisol deficiency. This impairs carbohydrate metabolism and other processes such as the action of catecholamines as pressor agents. Cortisol deficiency also stimulates ACTH secretion, causing adrenal hyperplasia.

21-OH deficiency also causes a build up of precursor steroids and therefore overproduction of steroids in other pathways (dehydroepiandrosterone [DHEA]→androstenedione→testosterone). This can cause virilization in female infants and therefore early diagnosis. In male infants there are no discernible effects, leading to later diagnosis.

CAH is categorized into 3 clinical forms depending on severity of defect: salt-wasting, simple virilization (no clinical signs of salt-wasting), and nonclassic (patients who come to attention as adolescent or adult females with virilism, acne, and menstrual irregularity).

Once this patient's CAH screening came back abnormal, it is important to confirm the diagnosis immediately. We must find out if there is an accumulation of 17-OH progesterone, and if so, is this patient salt-wasting, which is very serious. This patient's sodium was 126 and potassium 7.1. Without the positive newborn screening, this infant (since a male [because both testicles palpated]) probably would have presented with a seizure or be in shock.

Acute treatment consists of fluid replacement with saline solutions and administration of IV hydrocortisone. Long-term treatment consists of hydrocortisone and since this patient is a salt-loser, mineralocorticoid replacement (fluorocortisol).

476. Answer: D

The answer is Turner syndrome. Although webbed neck and coarctation of the aorta are classically described as features of Turner syndrome (TS), they are not the most common. Webbed neck only occurs in 25% and coarctation <20%. Bicuspid aortic valve occurs in up to 50%. Other common features besides those mentioned in this patient include complete gonadal failure, infertility, cubitus valgus, genu valgum, and renal abnormalities. Incidence of Hashimoto thyroiditis is also increased.

TS is caused by complete or partial X chromosome monosomy and is diagnosed by chromosomal karyotype. Treatment includes estrogen/progesterone replacement, and although these patients are not generally growth hormone deficient, growth hormone will accelerate growth and increase final height.

477. Answer: A

The correct answer is change IVF to 5% glucose in 0.2% NaCl with added potassium. Diabetic ketoacidosis (DKA) must be treated with insulin and fluid/electrolyte correction. Patients in DKA are in a hyperosmolar state due to the hyperglycemia so even 0.9% (isotonic) saline is hypotonic compared to the patient's serum osmolality. It is imperative to slowly decrease the patient's osmolality because too rapid a decline can cause cerebral edema. Initial fluid bolus given should be 0.9% saline followed by 0.45% saline with potassium. Potassium shifts from extracellular to intracellular during correction of acidosis; therefore, if potassium is not given, severe hypokalemia could result. As blood glucose levels approach 300 mg/dL, 5% glucose (added to 0.2% saline with added potassium) is started to limit the decline in osmolality and reduce the risk of cerebral edema.

478. Answer: D

The correct answer is physiologic pubertal gynecomastia. This is a very common condition (about 2/3) during early to mid puberty. The cause is not fully understood but is believed to be caused by an estrogen-androgen imbalance. The gynecomastia can be either unilateral or bilateral. Tenderness is common but transitory. Spontaneous regression can occur within a few months to 2 years. Treatment consists of reassurance to family.

479. Answer: E

The correct answer is the presence or absence of specific ossification centers as compared to known standards. Remember that crazy book in radiology? You stared and stared at it but just saw a bunch of bones--but the radiologist and the endocrinologist stood there and argued over whether the child is 8 years and 1 month versus 8 years and 5 weeks! Usually this occurred during your important scheduled lunch-time lecture—ok, I'm regressing back to residency.

480. Answer: B

The correct answer is follows the maximal growth in height. This kinda makes sense—Think of the tall, lanky kid who you see all the time. He has just finished his height spurt and the next time you see him he looks like Arnold—bulked up and muscular—it doesn't happen the other way around—they don't bulk up and then get tall. For those of you who went for "age 40" answer—I'm with you—but alas this is the pediatrics Boards and not a "Fantasy Island" episode.

481. Answer: D

The correct answer is darkly pigmented, slightly curly pubic hair. Remember, in women, pubic hair and breast development are the only things that determine Tanner staging! So you should have thrown out the acne and menarche right away—they occur in puberty but don't determine Tanner Staging. The breast mound is seen in Tanner 2 and the light pubic hair is seen in Tanner 2 also. Tanner 3 has the development of dark, curly pubic hair.

482. Answer: E

The correct answer is the bone age is usually normal or only slightly delayed. In these children, slow linear growth is noted in early childhood. The growth curve is actually on a normal parallel with the normal growth curve. However, the curve usually is just below or near the bottom of the normal curve. Ultimate height is below average (why else would they call it short stature??). The onset of puberty is not delayed and follows age norms.

483. Answer: B

The correct answer is they show slowing of growth velocity and fall off the normal growth curve. Bone age is generally delayed. Since this is an "isolated" growth hormone deficiency, no other abnormality is found as far as the endocrine system. You need to check for craniopharyngioma or associated pituitary abnormality such as ACTH deficiency or both before you can say "this is an isolated growth hormone deficiency".

484. Answer: A

The correct answer is she will likely be normal height and weight. Children with delayed puberty are initially short but have a longer than normal period of growth and a later than normal adolescent growth spurt. So, in the end she will likely be normal for both height and weight.. (so much for your season passes..).

485. Answer: B

The correct answer is following menarche by 12 to 24 months. MOST do this. (We all know the 12 or 13 year-old kid who comes in pregnant and says they never had menses). Also, in young teens who are sexually active—they may get a "surprise" after having sex for 2 years without contraception—because they haven't ovulated until the most recent sexual encounter.

486. Answer: D

The correct answer is it usually occurs at the same time as Tanner stages 4 to 5. Menarche usually follows rather than precedes the adolescent growth spurt. Usually, menarche means that the adolescent growth spurt is over and there is little further increase in height.

487. Answer: A

The correct answer is craniopharyngioma. This tumor is often associated with hypothalamic and pituitary destruction and dysfunction—this may present in later childhood or adolescence as growth failure. A sudden arrest of growth should raise suspicion for this diagnosis. The severity of this growth change pretty much rules out normal variant or constitutional growth delay. Androgen excess can lead to ultimate short stature—initially however, it would lead to accelerated growth in height and the child would be tall for his age initially.

488. Answer: D

The correct "incorrect" answer is Cushing's syndrome. Cushing's syndrome results in glucocorticoid excess. This leads to WEIGHT gain but retardation in linear growth. Soto's syndrome is cerebral gigantism and mental retardation. Exogenous growth hormone, if given to a child, could result in excessive growth. Marfan's is associated with tall stature. Virilizing adrenal tumors present with excessive growth velocities—however if the tumors accelerate epiphyseal plate closure then the child could be of final short stature.

489. Answer: E

The correct "incorrect" answer is measuring urinary VMA is likely to be helpful. The leading diagnosis is a partial 21-hydroxylase deficiency—this would result in diminished cortisol production, which would stimulate increased ACTH output—this restores cortisol production to normal but results in a HUGE increase in the production of androgens and cortisol precursors. Thus, measuring plasma levels of 17-hydroxyprogeserone and urinary levels of 17-ketosteroids would be diagnostic. Excess cortisol explains the weight but not the height, as cortisol inhibits linear growth. The presence of normal testes argues against excess gonadotropins.

490. Answer: D

The correct answer is the penis, testes, and scrotum have all enlarged considerably and are approaching adult size. The pubic hair at this stage is limited to the pubic area and does not extend onto the medial thighs or linea alba until stage 5. Males reach Tanner stage 5 at an average age of 14 with a range of 12 to 16 ½ years.

491. Answer: D

The correct answer is Klinefelter's syndrome. A male who has "disjointed" Tanner stages—particularly where pubic hair is progressing but scrotal and testes size are not, should be evaluated for Klinefelter's. Other things to think about are conditions of excessive adrenal androgen secretion—or anabolic steroids in a high school athlete.

492. Answer: A

The correct answer is menarche usually begins before or during stage 4. ¼ will have menarche in Tanner stage 3 and 60% will have menarche during Tanner stage 4. That only leaves 15% to have menarche in Tanner stage 5. Tanner stage 4 breast development consists of projection of both areola and papilla to form a distinct, secondary mound above the level of the breast. In stage 5, the areola is recessed to the general contour of the breast, so only the papilla projects.

493. Answer: D

The correct answer is check serum IGF-1 and 24-hour urine cortisol. Whenever a pituitary incidentaloma is discovered, two main questions must be answered. One, is the mass inhibiting secretion of any pituitary tumors. Two, is the tumor secreting something. Let's review the inhibiting scenario first. Many pituitary tumors do not appear to secrete anything and are called null cell tumors. With the advent of sensitive assays, it has been learned that some of these null-cell tumors actually do secrete. They may be secreting α-chains or gonadotrophins (LH or FSH), which rarely cause symptoms. After all, which man is going to complain about larger testes or a higher sperm count. However, some of these tumors get large enough that they inhibit secretion of pituitary hormones because of a mass-effect. In this patient, the tumor is a microadenoma (< 10 mm) and is too small to inhibit secretion.

The other scenario is one of excess secretion. Does the pituitary tumor secrete any hormones? Remember the main 6 anterior pituitary hormones: ACTH, LH, FSH, GH, TSH, PRL. A fishing expedition to test all hormones is not recommended. Instead, evaluate the patient for signs or symptoms that may point towards a particular excess such as galactorrhea or loss of libido (PRL); amenorrhea (LH, FSH); weight loss, hyperdefecation, tachyarrhythmia, heat intolerance (TSH); hypertension, hypokalemia, alkalosis (ACTH). These findings can be very subtle or even absent in the case of a new tumor or a very small one. If your evaluation does not point toward a particular hormone, then check the adrenal and thyroid axes. A screening test for the adrenal axis is a 24-hour urine for cortisol and a value < 70 µg is normal. The thyroid axis can be checked by a TSH and T4 drawn at any time of the day. I must caution you to check one more hormone. A small tumor may be secreting GH. The effects of over-secretion of GH takes many years to become evident and many more years usually transpire before it is recognized. These patients develop acromegaly and its many serious complications. Though GH is pulsatile, its effect on IGF-1 is not. Measure a random IGF-1 in any patient with a pituitary incidentaloma. In this patient, the central obesity and hypertension may indicate hypercortisolism (Cushing's syndrome). Order a 24-hour urine for cortisol and don't forget to check the IGF-1 level.

"Refer him to a neurosurgeon for transsphenoidal resection of the pituitary mass" is incorrect because there are no reasons to refer this patient for surgery at this time.
"Return to your clinic in a few weeks to recheck blood pressure" is incorrect because the pituitary tumor must be evaluated and his blood pressure management must be followed. "Discharge him from your clinic on a drug to treat hypertension and encourage him to stop riding motorcycles" is incorrect because, once again, the pituitary tumor must be evaluated. "Check an ACTH stimulation test, TSH, and a total testosterone" is incorrect because hyposecretion of ACTH, secondary hypothyroidism, and secondary hypogonadism are not suspected.

494. Answer: E

The correct answer is the patient probably does not have any thyroid problems. This patient is critically sick. In severe illness, the pituitary secretes less TSH which results in a low or low-normal FT4. However, T4 is not the active hormone; T3 is active. In severe illness, T3 levels are greatly suppressed. With the T4 being lower, there is less T4 available to be converted into T3. However, there is still considerable T4 present. In order to protect the body from the active T3 hormone, the T4 is converted into an inactive hormone called reverse T3 (rT3). Levels of rT3 are rarely measured, but if it was measured in this patient, it would be greatly elevated.

This patient is most likely euthyroid, but very sick. He does not have hypothyroidism or hyperthyroidism, either primary or secondary. There is no need to treat his abnormal thyroid tests, other than to treat his underlying illness.

495. Answer: B

The correct answer is refer him for a thyroid fine needle biopsy and aspiration (FNA). This patient is euthyroid, but with a thyroid nodule. In children and adolescents there is a MUCH higher risk of cancer than in adults!! Some might even recommend a complete removal of the nodule because the risk of carcinoma is much more likely in children. The correct answer is to perform a thyroid FNA, either yourself or refer him to someone who can. If the biopsy is not conclusive, then repeat it. If the second biopsy is also inconclusive, then refer him to a surgeon for a hemithyroidectomy. A near-total thyroidectomy would only be needed if cancer was present. Many physicians in the past have tried to shrink nodules with thyroxine thinking that exogenous thyroxine will lower the TSH which will reduce the growth stimulation to the nodule. Unfortunately, studies have shown this not to be the case; thyroxine should not be given in the hope of shrinking a nodule. Considering how easy and safe a thyroid biopsy is, it would be inappropriate to just follow him. Though the vast majority of nodules are benign, cancer cannot be excluded by simply watching the nodule.

496. Answer: B

The correct answer is order TSH and FT4, suspecting hypothyroidism due to postpartum thyroiditis. Many young mothers will report postpartum depression which will resolve on its own. However, some of these cases of postpartum depression may actually signify postpartum thyroiditis. The typical presentation is an uneventful pregnancy and delivery followed by an initial period of hyperthyroidism lasting for about one month which is followed by a protracted period of hypothyroidism lasting for many months and sometimes for a year. The initial period of hyperthyroidism is easily tolerated. After all, the woman will have considerable energy and will more easily lose weight. However, she will soon develop hypothyroidism. Once you verify with TSH and FT4 that she is hypothyroid, begin treating her with thyroxine. Her hyperthyroidism is not likely to be permanent, so follow her monthly and adjust the thyroxine dose as needed, ultimately discontinuing it.

497. Answer: E

The correct answer is he has diabetes and must talk with a diabetes educator and dietitian to begin a diet and exercise program. He fulfills two diagnostic criteria for the diagnosis of diabetes. The full set of criteria include (1) random glucose ≥ 200 mg/dL with symptoms (polyuria, polydipsia, or unexplained weight loss), (2) fasting glucose ≥ 126 mg/dL, and (3) 2-hour 75 g oral glucose tolerance test (OGTT) ≥ 200 mg/dL. Now that you have diagnosed him with diabetes, you must next determine whether he has type 1 or type 2 diabetes. He most likely has type 2 because he is overweight and there is no mention of metabolic decompensation. You must now determine whether to treat and, if so, how to treat his diabetes. There is no question about it; you must intervene immediately. There is nothing to benefit from waiting. However, in the absence of metabolic decompensation and severe hyperglycemia, it is most prudent to begin with lifestyle changes. He must be educated on the importance of an exercise program (walking is usually enough) and he must learn how to eat a healthy diet. Diet and exercise may be all that he needs. Only if he fails such a regimen should he be started on drug therapy.

498. Answer: B

The correct answer is stop taking the metformin and to come to your office tomorrow. It is important to know the contraindications for use of metformin. Of course it is absolutely contraindicated when the patient has a known hypersensitivity to it or any component of the drug, but also in men with a creatinine ≥ 1.5 mg/dL or in women with a creatinine ≥ 1.4 mg/dL. This is a very commonly used drug and these numbers must be memorized for proper patient care. It is not unreasonable to be expected to know these numbers for the Boards. It is also important to know that relative contraindications include kidney, liver, and heart dysfunction.

He has good glycemic control and does not need a second agent at this time. There is no compelling reason to add a thiazolidinedione. The recommended LDL goal in a diabetic is < 100 mg/dL. His LDL is currently at goal and does not need a statin drug. In light of his creatinine level of 1.5 mg/dL, it is inappropriate to simply have him return to your clinic in 6 months. The blood pressure goal for a diabetic without albuminuria is < 130/80. His blood pressure is not elevated and he does not need to start any blood pressure lowering agents at this time.

499. Answer: A

The correct answer is to reduce her evening NPH insulin to 20 units and follow closely. You would decrease the evening insulin even further if the symptoms do not improve. Her symptoms of vivid nightmares and waking in a cold sweat are compatible with nocturnal hypoglycemia. The most likely explanation for the early morning hyperglycemia is that the nocturnal hypoglycemia is causing the contrainsular hormones (glucagon, cortisol, growth hormone, and epinephrine) to be secreted. Many type 1 diabetics lose the ability to secrete glucagon in response to hypoglycemia, but the remaining hormones are unaffected. These hormones will raise the glucose level. However, insulin deficient persons such as this patient do not have the ability to make their own insulin to control the hyperglycemic effect of the contrainsular hormones and her morning fasting glucose levels are elevated. Every patient taking insulin needs to perform self-monitoring of their blood glucose levels. They should check their glucose before and two hours after every meal, at bedtime, and in the middle of the night around 3 am. Of course it's impractical to constantly check glucose levels this often on a daily basis. One alternative is to have the patient check their glucose level twice every day, choosing different times each day so that the log book will have some numbers at each time point. The 3 am glucose level should be checked at least once each month, but doesn't need to be checked much more frequently unless the patient is having evidence of nocturnal hypoglycemia or has changed the insulin regimen. Once this patient no longer has hypoglycemia, the insulin can always be carefully and slowly increased.

It is inappropriate to begin an anxiolytic rather than decreasing the insulin. Hypoglycemia can be life-threatening. Increasing her evening insulin further could be fatal. There is no evidence that she has insulin resistance in addition to her insulin deficiency and adding an insulin sensitizer is inappropriate. Switching her to a 70/30 premix is also inappropriate. The goal of treating a type 1 diabetic is to replace the insulin in a physiologic way. Her insulin regimen is already physiologic by offering basal coverage with NPH twice daily and bolus coverage with a rapid-acting insulin analog with each meal.

500. Answer: A

The correct diagnosis is primary hyperparathyroidism. The PTH is elevated along with the calcium. Normally, an elevated calcium would suppress the PTH level. His PTH is elevated in the face of hypercalcemia and thus represents primary hyperparathyroidism.

His vitamin D levels are elevated, but this is due to both his primary hyperparathyroidism and his use of vitamin supplements. Vitamin A intoxication can cause hypercalcemia, but no vitamin A levels are given in this question and his primary hyperparathyroidism is a better explanation. Pseudopseudohypoparathyroidism refers to a specific phenotype (shortened 4th and 5th metacarpals) with normal calcium and parathyroid hormone levels. His labs rule out such a diagnosis. Secondary hyperparathyroidism refers to the normally elevated levels of parathyroid hormone in the face of hypocalcemia. Low calcium levels will stimulate the parathyroid glands to secrete extra hormone which will stimulate the conversion of 25OH-vitamin D into 1,25(OH)$_2$-vitamin D. His calcium is elevated and thus he cannot have secondary hyperparathyroidism.

501. Answer: D

The correct answer is Vitamin D deficiency. This girl has probably had hypocalcemia for quite some time and only came to medical attention because she experienced an osteoporotic hip fracture. An extremely common cause of hypocalcemia is vitamin D deficiency and she exhibits a classic presentation. Her 25OH-Vitamin D level is low, reflecting both her poor diet and her low exposure to sunlight. Hypocalcemia normally gives rise to an elevated parathyroid hormone level (secondary hyperparathyroidism) and this in turn stimulates the conversion of 25OH-Vitamin D to $1,25(OH)_2$-Vitamin D. Unfortunately, her levels of 25OH-Vitamin D are already low and her conversion to $1,25(OH)_2$-Vitamin D is thus impaired. The phosphate level is low because of the hyperparathyroidism which stimulates renal excretion of phosphates.

While hypomagnesemia can cause hypocalcemia due to impaired secretion of the parathyroid hormone, her hypermagnesemia is not contributing. Hyperphosphatemia may cause hypocalcemia because of local precipitation of calcium-phosphate salts. Her hypophosphatemia is not the cause of the hypocalcemia. Thiazide diuretics are associated with hypercalcemia, not hypocalcemia. Primary hyperparathyroidism causes hypercalcemia, not hypocalcemia.

502. Answer: C

The correct answer is dopamine agonist. Whenever a girl or woman has not had menses, exclude pregnancy.   DO NOT forget this test in any patient with abdominal pain…ruptured ectopic pregnancy is a favorite Board question as is ruptured spleen, but I digress. Severe hypothyroidism (i.e. with TSH over 50) can cause pituitary enlargement and hyperprolactinemia that resolve with thyroxine administration. If the TSH is markedly elevated, there is no need for a T4 or the other serum tests. Because the prolactin level is below 100-200, your suspicion for co-secretory or an extremely large pituitary adenoma interrupting the dopamine inhibitory paths in the pituitary stalk, should be high and therefore you should obtain the additional tests. Prolactinomas can co-secrete human growth hormone (hGH). The treatment of acromegaly with prolactinoma is surgical so it must be excluded. Hopefully, this degree of sophistication will not be expected for the Boards…remember it in practice, however. MRI gives the best sella definition especially as she may have a very small prolactinoma. Excluding Cushing's disease is important because it causes menstrual disruption and can be the first recognized symptom. If she has a large pituitary tumor, the T4 would be low due to inadequate TSH-secretory reserve.   Do NOT forget medication history in all clinical case questions. The physiology that the hyperprolactinemic state disrupts is ovarian cycling: therefore, infertility, and low estrogen state with potential for endometrial hyperplasia (as the progesterone surge and its consequent endometrial deciduation is suppressed), osteopenia, and loss of estrogen's cardio protection. If the tumor enlarges sufficiently it can cause visual field loss. This is one time when anatomy becomes as important as FUNCTION in endocrine evaluation.

503. Answer: A

The correct "incorrect" answer is Headache. Pituitary tumors are secretory and hyperplasia of all the cell types has been reported: TSH, ACTH, hGH, Gonadotrophins and prolactin. Through mass effect, a nonsecretory or secretory adenoma can cause deficiency in the production of the other hormones, especially TSH and ACTH. In adolescents and young adults, headache is almost never caused by, or when present, relieved by treatment for a pituitary adenoma.

504. Answer: C

The correct answer is Cortrosyn stimulation. This is a classic presentation for Addison's disease. She has fatigue, asthenia and listlessness and recurrent flu-like illnesses. Further history may be that of a family history of autoimmune endocrine disorders (Type 1 Diabetes, Hashimoto's disease, Grave's disease) or of tuberculosis she acquired overseas if it had been left untreated…but that is too convoluted for the Boards. The Cortrosyn stimulation is the diagnostic test and should be done next. Screening for other autoimmune endocrine disorders is reasonable, but not a priority. This is not the history of bulimia so a dental screening for enamel etching due to vomiting is lower on the list. Treatment should be a corticosteroid and mineralocorticoid as the aldosterone-producing cells are often involved to some extent.

505. Answer: B

The correct answer is Klinefelter's syndrome. This exam points toward eunuchoid development with span greater than height, which is compatible with late epiphyseal closure due to underproduction of testosterone, the gynecomastia also points toward relative insufficient testosterone production. The key is the small (usually described as firm) testes and gynecomastia, which point to Klinefelter's syndrome. Kallmann's syndrome: congenital hypogonadotrophic hypogonadism has low amounts of both estrogens and testosterone so gynecomastia does not develop.

506. Answer: E

The correct answer is to increase the supper Humalog and decrease the bedtime NPH. You are asked to recognize that erratic fasting glucoses may represent unrecognized nocturnal hypoglycemia, and cut her bedtime NPH.

507. Answer: A

The correct answer is symptoms of hypoglycemia, low serum glucose, and symptom relief with glucose. This question asks you to understand causes of hypoglycemia, and differentiate between fasting (insulinoma) and post-prandial (dumping syndrome and "reactive") hypoglycemia. Once you discriminate between hypoglycemia which occurs in the fasting state which is due to insulin excess—endogenous or exogenous and that which occurs after eating, the correct diagnosis is post-gastrectomy syndrome. Also it is necessary to remember that Whipple's triad of hypoglycemic symptoms occurs during periods of low serum glucose and is relieved by a source of sugar.

508. Answer: E

The correct "incorrect" answer is growth hormone concentration = 0.2 micrograms/L 1 hour after oral administration of 100 g glucose (NL = suppression below 1 micrograms/L). Growth hormone concentration should NOT be suppressed in his condition which is Growth Hormone Excess. He presents with the clinical syndrome of acromegaly with bony and soft tissue overgrowth, enlargement of the jaw and tongue, wide spacing of the teeth, and coarsened facial features. Hypertension may result because of expansion of the plasma volume and total body sodium. A moist, oily, doughy handshake is characteristic.

Laboratory findings include abnormal glucose tolerance and mild hyperprolactinemia. The reason for growth hormone excess in almost all patients with acromegaly is a pituitary adenoma. Useful screening tests include measurements of glucose-suppressed growth hormone concentrations (which normally is suppressed to below 1 microgram/L) and IGF binding protein 3. IGF-I concentrations are elevated secondary to the high levels of growth hormone. Once you have confirmed acromegaly or have a good suspicion, you should proceed to MRI to find the pituitary adenoma.

509. Answer: B

The correct "incorrect" answer is Graves disease. You were thinking all along it was Graves right? Well that stupid radioactive iodine uptake test threw that answer out—with Graves it is never LOW. The thyrotoxic phase of subacute and silent thyroiditis is associated with an inflammatory breakdown and release of stored thyroid hormone, which will feed back onto the hypothalamus and anterior pituitary to inhibit TSH secretion. This will produce a low RAIU for a while. Struma ovarii remember, consists of ectopic hyperfunctioning autonomous thyroid tissue—like in a teratoma which also will result in a low RAIU in the thyroid (when the pelvis is scanned though it would show an INCREASED uptake here). Iodine-induced thyrotoxicosis will generally occur in the face of a preexisting dysfunctional thyroid. We see this mainly in someone who is coming from a country with low iodine intake and then they come to the great USA with our HIGH iodine intakes.

510. Answer: E

The correct answer is to do nothing at this point. This guy has Familial Hypocalciuric Hypercalcemia (FHH) also known as benign familial hypercalcemia. This consists of an elevated serum calcium, normal or low serum phosphorus, a normal or high serum PTH, a slightly elevated magnesium and a low urinary calcium excretion. This is inherited as an autosomal dominant disorder of chromosomes 3 or 19. No therapy is required—remember a favorite of the ABP—to do as little as possible.

Surgery will not correct the hypercalcemia. The other thing to be careful about is that these patients can be misdiagnosed with hyperparathyroidism if the urinary calcium is not measured. Untreated, these patients generally remain asymptomatic without evidence of renal calculi, HTN, or other problems with hypercalcemia.

511. Answer: D

The correct answer is radioactive iodine uptake. This post partum female has symptoms and lab work suggesting hyperthyroidism. The most common cause in this setting would be post partum thyroiditis. The most definitive test to rule out the alternative diagnosis of Grave's disease would be a 24 hour radioactive iodine uptake. Patients with Grave's disease have a high 24 hour radioiodine uptake, whereas patients with acute or subacute thyroiditis have a very low radioiodine uptake.

512. Answer: A

The correct answer is 3_β-hydroxysteroid dehydrogenase. Ambiguous genitalia in association with congenital adrenal hyperplasia usually means a female pseudohermaphrodite—because most of the defects result in masculinization of the baby. However, this patient is 46 XY and a genetic male. The rare defect of 3_β-hydroxysteroid dehydrogenase causes an inability to synthesize testicular androgen and therefore failure of normal masculinization of the male baby—(think Richard Simmons!). The 17-hydroxylase can cause feminization but it is NOT associated with salt loss. So to figure this question out—You have a MALE with ambiguous genitalia—so he must have undergone feminization.

513. Answer: C

The correct answer is bone age. Premature thelarche is a benign condition of isolated breast development in girls under 8-years-old without other signs of sexual maturation. It is caused by increased bioactivity at the level of breast tissue. Breast tissue is extremely sensitive to estrogen which explains why other estrogen-sensitive tissues are unaffected. Key features include isolated breast development without other secondary sexual characteristics, normal linear growth, and normal skeletal maturation. Therefore the only test needed is a bone age to exclude progressive forms of precocious puberty. If bone age is age-appropriate or delayed, no further tests are needed. If advanced, referral to an endocrinologist and possible pelvic ultrasound are warranted. Measurements of FSH, LH, and estradiol are usually not helpful. Observation is usually sufficient.

514. Answer: A

The correct answer is brain tumors are the most common *solid* tumors in children. They are surpassed only by leukemia as the most common *neoplasm* in children. Tumors in children are usually infratentorial (cerebellar, 4th ventricle, brain stem) and usually are midline (3rd and 4th ventricles, optic chiasm, and brainstem). Acoustic neuromas, meningiomas, and pituitary adenomas are more common in adults. Optic gliomas and craniopharyngiomas are more common in children.

515. Answer: C

The correct answer is chiasmal compression by tumor—of which the most likely would be a craniopharyngioma, chiasmal glioma, teratoma, or other tumor in the chiasmal area. None of the other conditions would give you this finding on physical examination.

516. Answer: A

The correct answer is of the posterior fossa tumors in children, medulloblastoma is the most frequent. It is more common in boys and the peak incidence is between 3 and 5 years of age. Seizures are relatively uncommon with this tumor. The tumor is very radiosensitive but the tumor seeds the entire neuroaxis. The onset of symptoms is fairly rapid and acute when compared to astrocytomas.

517. Answer: C

The correct answer is most likely will be mentally retarded and may develop seizures. This patient has Rett syndrome which is a neurodegenerative disorder of unknown etiology that occurs in female children. They have normal development until approximately 1 year of age at which time they show regression of language and motor skills. Deceleration of head growth begins between 2-4 months of age resulting in acquired microcephaly. The hallmark of Rett syndrome is repetitive hand wringing movements with loss of purposeful hand movement.

In infancy these children may be irritable and have failure of head growth. The toddler age demonstrates hypotonia and regression of language and cerebration. In children ages 2-10 years, mental retardation becomes apparent and one-third of cases develop seizures. Most patients survive to adulthood although there is an unexplained increased risk of sudden death during sleep in the first 2 decades.

MRI shows a decrease in brain volume and slight increase in the size of the ventricles. There is no specific treatment available. Treatment of seizures is effective using standard anticonvulsants.

518. Answer: B

The correct answer is Guillain-Barré syndrome. Guillain-Barré is the most common inflammatory polyneuropathy. It frequently is preceded by an upper respiratory infection and has been associated with *Campylobacter jejuni* infections as well as EBV, CMV, HIV, Mycoplasma, and Lyme disease. Symptoms include an ASCENDING paralysis and AREFLEXIA caused by a segmental demyelination of the peripheral nerves. CSF examination can be helpful and may show an elevated protein with a small increase in CSF WBCs. Nerve conduction studies show slowed conduction. Plasmapheresis is useful if it is begun early in the course.

Botulism causes a DESCENDING paralysis and begins with CRANIAL nerve weakness manifested by dysphonia, dysphagia, diplopia, and blurred vision, then followed by the muscle weakness and respiratory insufficiency. Poliomyelitis presents as meningeal symptoms, fever, and asymmetric paralysis. Tick paralysis occurs while the tick is attached and is due to a neurotoxin. It causes an ascending flaccid paralysis and ataxia. Rabies would not be associated with these types of neurologic findings.

519. Answer: D

The correct answer is ceftriaxone and vancomycin. She has pneumococcal meningitis. Realize that in many parts of the United States, up to 30% of pneumococci are resistant to penicillin and up to 10% are resistant to the 3rd generation cephalosporins. Know that Vancomycin and ceftriaxone are appropriate for presumed pneumococcal meningitis until the sensitivities are known. Another option is ceftriaxone and rifampin. Her prior antibiotic usage increases her risk of having a resistant organism. Ceftazidime is a poor choice as it has diminished gram-positive activity compared to ceftriaxone and cefotaxime. Penicillin alone would be a poor choice because of the high resistant rates. Now, if they tell you the pneumococcus is sensitive to penicillin then that would be the correct choice!

520. Answer: A

The correct answer is Herpes simplex meningoencephalitis. The key here is the "bizarre behavior" and the findings on MRI of temporal lobe involvement. To help you diagnose this, a PCR for Herpes simplex virus DNA could be helpful on the CSF. CSF cultures for herpes are rarely positive except in the severely immunocompromised or in neonates. He certainly is at risk for syphilis (past urethritis and an adolescent) but the CSF findings don't support it nor does the MRI. You would though order a CSF VDRL on this kid just because he is at high risk based on his past history. *Bartonella henselae* is the etiology for Cat Scratch disease and does cause significant CNS disease in children on occasion—it is more commonly associated with seizures. Seizures also are likely with Herpes encephalitis too. We have no indication he has varicella and this does not look like bacterial meningitis with the normal protein and glucose.

521. Answer: C

The correct answer is Duchenne muscular dystrophy (DMD). It is a degenerative genetic disorder caused by a defect located at the p21 location on the X chromosome. It is the most common muscular dystrophy presenting in childhood. The age of onset is between 2-6 years with difficulty climbing stairs, Gower's maneuver, and falling. This is followed by a Trendelenburg gait. The patient loses the ability to ambulate between 10-12 years of age. Pseudohypertrophy of calves and cardiomyopathy are also features of the disease. Death usually occurs by age 20. CPK is extremely elevated and muscle biopsy shows variation in fiber size, connective tissue proliferation, type IIB fiber deficiency, and absent dystrophin. This is differentiated from Becker muscular dystrophy (BMD) in that patients with BMD have later onset in childhood (5-10 years old) with death usually occurring in their late 20s. Muscle biopsy findings are similar except type IIB fibers and dystrophin are present.

522. Answer: B

The correct answer is child abuse. External signs of trauma are frequently missing if the trauma is due to shaking. Always look for retinal hemorrhages if they ask you about this on the Boards! Common signs in an infant to think about retinal hemorrhages are lethargy, irritability, and vomiting—the same things to be worried about with regard to sepsis. Also, failure to thrive can occur in abused children too—so be on the look out for that. In severe cases, coma, seizures and focal neurologic signs can occur.

523. Answer: D

The correct answer is craniopharyngioma. Increased intracranial pressure and x-ray findings of calcifications in the region of the sella turcica are common findings in children with craniopharyngiomas. Visual defects (due to involvement of the optic chiasm or optic nerve) and endocrine dysfunction are also common. The most common endocrine dysfunction is growth failure due to involvement of the pituitary gland.

524. Answer: B

The correct answer is Werdnig-Hoffman disease. She has all of the classic findings. Suspect it in a child under 2 years of age who has progressive weakness with tongue fasciculations!

525. Answer: D

The correct answer is spastic. Nearly ¾ of cases of cerebral palsy are of the spastic type. Most commonly hemiplegia or quadriplegia is seen. Findings include increased muscle tone, increased deep tendon reflexes, clonus and present Babinski reflexes.

526. Answer: A

The correct answer is acute cerebellitis. This is an acute, short-lived inflammation of the cerebellum and is usually viral or postinfectious in etiology. The prognosis is excellent and improvement usually occurs rapidly within a week. With the normal CT scan, posterior fossa tumor is unlikely. The abnormal CSF with WBCs is helpful in dismissing alcohol, Hartnup's disease as well as other potential toxins. Neuroblastoma would be rare without other symptoms.

527. Answer: C

The correct answer is hyper-alertness, euphoria, and severe failure to thrive. The syndrome is usually due to a lesion, commonly a glioma, in the region of the hypothalamus. The syndrome is only seen in infants—if older children or adults get tumors in this area they develop obesity.

528. Answer: B

The correct answer is craniosynostosis plus extensive syndactyly of the fingers and toes. This is an autosomal dominant syndrome.

529. Answer: E

The correct "incorrect" answer is recurrent *Streptococcus* pharyngitis. Cystic fibrosis probably is associated with increased incidence due to extension from sinuses; but some speculate that hypoxia and pulmonary artery-to-vein shunting may play a role also. Cerebral hypoxia may cause focal encephalomalacia, predisposing to infection. Right-to-left cardiac shunts bypass the macrophage-filtering mechanism of the lung and increase the ability for bacteria to reach the brain. Obviously penetration of the brain by a foreign object is likely to introduce infection—DUH? Chronic otitis media and other infections may predispose via direct extension and occasionally via bacteremia.

530. Answer: B

The correct answer is 4 months. Remember that initially infants have a "grasp reflex" that disappears between 2 and 3 months. The ability to VOLUNTARILY grasp something usually occurs between the ages of 2 and 4 months—by 4 months 90% of infants are able to grasp a rattle voluntarily. Can you grasp this?

531. Answer: B

The correct answer is circle (at 2 ½ to 3 ½ years), cross (3 ½ to 4 ½ years) and square (5 to 6 years). These are fine-motor adaptive characteristics and develop in regular order.

532. Answer: C

The correct answer is 125 mg/dl. The concentration gradually falls to less than 45 mg/dl by 6 to 8 weeks of age.

533. Answer: C

The correct answer is fully understandable but frequently speaks with mispronunciations and grammatical errors. First, the question writer is from Louisiana—so he knows what he is talking about..but alas, the American Board of Pediatrics does not recognize Louisiana as a risk factor—actually I could put any State in there. If you want, put your state in the answer—you probably would agree even if you are from "sniff" Massachusetts—ok, ok…now I'll get those folk upset..I"ll stop while I'm ahead. Those mispronunciations and grammatical errors continue until the age of 5 (hmm..guess some of us never grow out of that one.)

534. Answer: C

The correct answer is 35 cm. A larger head at birth may indicate hydrocephalus or an intracranial bleed. Or, it could mean that the kid should grow up and work for a medical publishing company. A small head at birth may indicate microcephaly and all of the millions of things that can do that. These children could grow up and write questions for the American Board of Surgery.

535. Answer: B

The correct answer is 2.5 cm. A greater than normal increase in head circumference could indicate subdurals or hydrocephalus. Less than normal may indicated brain injury particularly from infection or trauma.

536. Answer: E

The correct answer is 3 to 4 years of age. If you have kids at home, try this—I swear it is the easiest way I can remember this stuff. My poor daughters were 3 and 1 when I took the Boards after residency. I think I did the Denver Developmental test on them like 100 times. They really got tired though of having to do that calculus work at bedtime…Oh yea back to the answer for this question— The kid should be able to copy a circle by 3. The cross drawing should occur sometime between 3 and 4. Copying a square won't happen until 4 to 5 years of age. So, if she can get the circle, she has to be older than 3. She can't do the square, which happens between 4 and 5. So she must be less than 4 and more than 3. Voila!

537. Answer: E

The correct answer is 2 months. ☺ This social tool is never lost—unless you frown all the time as an adult?

538. Answer: B

The correct answer is 3 months. The social laugh appears later than the social smile. About ½ of infants are able to have a social laugh by 2 months; 90% by 3 months. Some adults have a great social laugh! Come to a MedStudy Pediatrics Intensive Course—You'll hear the best social laugh in the world!

539. Answer: E

The correct answer is 7 months. 50% of normal children can sit alone without support by 5 ½ months and almost 90% can by 7 months.

540. Answer: D

The correct answer is 14 months. Unassisted walking is achieved usually sometime between 10 and 14 months; with 90% of kids being able to walk unassisted by that point.

541. Answer: A

The correct answer is 1 year. The ability to release an object in a controlled fashion is much more difficult than grasping at objects. Hmm..sometimes I wonder if my daughter has that ability with the credit card?

542. Answer: A

The correct answer is 2 years. About 50% of children can do it by 18 months of age. The majority can do it by the age of 2 years.

543. Answer: A

The correct answer is 5 months. Gosh darn...don't you just cringe when you see that "regard and reach for" phrase. How in the heck does a baby "regard" something? Who uses that verb?? Oh well. Just know it. Note that they just have to "reach for it" not actually grab it. The "grabbing part" won't occur in a majority of kids for a few months more or even later. That little raisin is hard to get unless you've got your "pincer" skills down.

544. Answer: E

The correct answer is all of the reflexes listed are "normal". Their absence in early infancy indicates a neurologic problem...their persistence into later childhood is also an indication of neurologic malfunction.

545. Answer: D

The correct "incorrect' answer is appears by 1 month of age. Usually it does not appear until 6 or 8 months of age. To do this one: You hold the baby by the waist and tilt or thrust him/her forward as if dropping him/her (obviously you don't drop the baby). A normal response is abduction and extension of the arms as if to break the fall—like crazy people who jump out of airplanes.

546. Answer: B

The correct answer is it is a spontaneous extension of the neck and spine with some stiffening of the lower extremities in response to being suspended prone by supporting the chest. It appears at about 6 months of age and persists until about 2 ½ years. That sounds hard enough on a 2 ½ year old kid. It is a higher level reflex. Do you really think someone would try this on a 10-year-old? Maybe if you were the Incredible Hulk and could pick up the kid with your palm?

547. Answer: D

The correct answer is it is a common finding in spastic cerebral palsy. This reflex is demonstrated with the infant supine. You extend both legs and then stroke the plantar aspect of each foot. A positive response consists of flexion of the OPPOSITE leg, followed by extension and abduction. It is normally present at birth and fades by 2 to 3 months of age. It is a spinal cord reflex.

548. Answer: A

The correct answer is CT scan without contrast. This patient has symptoms consistent with acute subarachnoid hemorrhage. He has sudden onset of a severe headache and no prior history of severe headaches. He is young though for this—the average age is about 45 years. The neck stiffness is due to meningeal irritation from blood. Blood in the subarachnoid space shows up very well on CT scan and contrast is NOT needed. Acute bleeds are better imaged by non-contrast CT scan than MRIs. The CT scan is a preferable first option over a lumbar puncture, because if the CT is positive, an LP would not be necessary.

549. Answer: E

The correct answer is no imaging. This patient has typical symptoms of migraine headaches. She is at a common age for the onset of migraines. Migraines are more common in women. The quality standards subcommittee of the American Academy of Neurology does not recommend the use of CNS imaging in adult patients with recurrent headaches typical of migraine, without focal neurologic signs or symptoms.

550. Answer: C

The correct answer is Head MRI. This girl has recurrent neurologic symptoms, with improvement between episodes. This history is suggestive of multiple sclerosis. The most sensitive imaging procedure for MS is MRI. Although lesions can occur in the spinal cord, the brain is the best first imaging site.

551. Answer: D

The correct answer is reaction to phenytoin. This patient is having a reaction to phenytoin, creating pseudolymphoma syndrome. He has fever, elevated transaminases, and generalized lymphadenopathy. A negative RPR effectively rules out secondary syphilis. He has no exposure history to suggest hepatitis B or Tularemia. Hodgkin's disease is a possibility, but the rapid onset and involvement of the liver, and diffuse lymphadenopathy would indicate advanced disease, less likely for such a rapid presentation.

552. Answer: E

The correct answer is none of the choices are likely. This patient has had headaches for six months. The most likely diagnosis is headache associated with oral contraceptive pills. She has a small risk for Pseudotumor cerebri, as she is obese. This diagnosis is excluded by the normal funduscopic exam. There are no cutaneous features suggestive of tuberous sclerosis (ash leaf spot, adenoma sebaceum).

553. Answer: C

The correct answer is amitriptyline. This kid is suffering from postherpetic neuralgia. Narcotics can also be used for treatment of postherpetic neuralgia-especially if the pain is severe. The anti-seizure medications gabapentin (Neurontin) and carbamazepine (Tegretol) are effective for postherpetic neuralgia. Phenytoin (Dilantin) and phenobarbital are not usually used because of toxicity and unproven efficacy.

554. Answer: A

The correct answer is Nylen-Bárány maneuver. This patient has very brief episodes of vertigo, which usually occur when he has a sudden change of position such as rolling over in bed. This is the classic description of benign positional vertigo. This diagnosis is confirmed clinically with the Nylen-Bárány maneuver (also called the Hallpike-Dix maneuver). The patient is rapidly moved from a seated position to one with the head hanging 45° below horizontal and rotated 45° to one side. The patient is observed for nystagmus. The maneuver is repeated toward the other side after the patient sits up. Movements have to be rapid. The nystagmus is sometimes quite subtle. In a peripheral lesion the latency of nystagmus or vertigo is 0-40 secs, duration is < 1 min, it fatigues with repeated testing, the direction of nystagmus is fixed and it is inconsistently reproduced. The nystagmus can be marked and the vertigo severe. There is no specific testing such as an audiogram ENG, or MRI that would make this diagnosis.

555. Answer: C

The correct answer is Cerumen impaction. This patient has noticed decreased hearing in his right ear. He has risk factors for hearing loss including recent treatment with aminoglycosides. The results of the Rinne test and Weber test are diagnostic in this case. The Rinne test shows air conduction louder than bone conduction in the left ear and bone conduction louder than air conduction in the right ear (symptomatic ear). This is consistent with a conductive hearing loss in his right ear. The Weber test confirms this bilateralizing to the ear with the conductive hearing loss. Aminoglycoside toxicity would cause a sensory hearing loss as would Acoustic neuroma and Ménière's disease and cochlear osteosclerosis. Unilateral cerumen impaction would cause a conductive hearing loss on the side of the impaction.

556. Answer: C

The correct answer is have patient call 911 for emergency evaluation /transport to ER. This patient has symptoms consistent with CO poisoning: headache, nausea ,vomiting, diarrhea and dyspnea. The key piece of clinical information is the improvement when he went outside to shovel snow. The appropriate management would be immediate removal from his home and immediate supportive care in an ER.

557. Answer: D

The correct answer is seizure (postictal). When confronted with a question like this, narrow the list first. Stroke is unlikely because of his age and the lack of focal neurologic findings. Encephalitis is unlikely without a fever and elevated white count. Hyperglycemia is out – the routine labs are negative. Drug intoxication is possible, as is a seizure/postictal state. Of these choices, seizure wins over drug intoxications because of the lack of findings on examination (*no* papillary abnormalities).

558. Answer: D

The correct answer is toxicology. Although several of the tests would probably be performed while the patient is in the ED, the Boards are looking for *a single, best answer*. Given that there is no evidence of trauma, and no focal neurological deficits, the CT and skull x-ray are unlikely to help. The lack of meningeal signs eliminates diagnoses like encephalitis and subarachnoid hemorrhage, so the lumbar puncture is less likely to help. An ABG might help if carbon monoxide (CO) poisoning were suspected; however, we are told that his room was well-ventilated. Also, CO poisoning occurs most often in persons who use petroleum-burning space heaters in the winter. Although we see no evidence of drug intoxication on exam, toxicology would be very helpful in this situation.

559. Answer: A

The correct answer is Cluster headache. The normal exam in combination with these symptoms describes cluster headache. For the exam, you must know the difference between each of the listed headaches.

560. Answer: E

The correct answer is that all of the choices are correct. All of the listed agents are effective in cluster headache.

561. Answer: D

The correct answer is abscess. In this case, the gradually worsening headaches after an invasive procedure strongly suggests an abscess. The fever and focal neurological deficits confirm this. Remember, the triad of fever, focal deficits, and headache means *abscess*. In a bacterial meningitis, there are usually no focal neurological deficits.

562. Answer: A

The correct answer is Ménière's disease. The most likely diagnosis is Ménière's. The triad of episodic vertigo, hearing loss, and tinnitus makes this diagnosis. In Benign Positional Vertigo, the person would not be expected to have hearing loss. Labyrinthitis and neuronitis are usually monophasic illnesses, likely due to a virus. Although stroke can cause vertigo, it is unlikely to be recurrent. In addition, stroke rarely causes vertigo by itself.

563. Answer: D

The correct answer is Multiple Sclerosis. The most likely diagnosis is multiple sclerosis (MS). The history of transient neurologic dysfunction (the blurred vision) strongly supports the diagnosis. The patient has an upper motor neuron disease (the increased reflexes and positive Babinski), so Cauda Equina Syndrome and Guillain-Barré are not possible. The symptoms only involve the left side, so transverse myelitis, which would cause a paraparesis, is not possible. Stroke is unlikely because the patient is young, without risk factors for stroke, and the symptoms have gradually worsened for ten days. She denies orthostatic hypotension.

564. Answer: C

The correct answer is Tensilon Test. This patient has a characteristic presentation of Myasthenia Gravis. The age of onset is between the second and fourth decades of life but 20% of patients have symptoms before the age of 20. Myasthenia is due to circulating polyclonal IgG autoantibodies (produced by B-lymphocytes) to the acetylcholine receptor. It is characterized by weakness which worsens with physical activity. In about 40% of cases, the presenting complaint is diplopia. Other common symptoms include dysarthria, dysphagia, and decreased range of facial movements. Limb and neck weakness is common. It is uncommon for the limbs to be affected without other symptoms. Medications such as D-penicillamine (once used to treat rheumatoid arthritis) can cause drug-induced myasthenia. If the drug is discontinued, the myasthenia-like syndrome resolves. Although TIA and stroke must be considered in the diagnosis, it is very unusual for ischemia to produce diplopia alone. Often, other neurological symptoms are present. Graves ophthalmopathy must always be considered when a patient has diplopia. Often, physical signs of Graves' disease, such as the Graves' stare, will suggest a diagnosis of thyroid disease.

The first diagnostic test is the Tensilon test. When clinical signs are present (not just subjective diplopia), the Tensilon test can confirm the clinical diagnosis. Tensilon (edrophonium) is a short-acting acetylcholinesterase inhibitor that acts to prolong the effects of acetylcholine at the postsynaptic neuromuscular junction. This will reverse the weakness transiently. A positive test then, would be improvement in clinical signs. A second test is the acetylcholine receptor antibody test. It is positive in 50% of patients with ocular myasthenia, and positive in 90% of patients with generalized myasthenia. In this case (ocular symptoms only), it would be a second line test. CT of the chest would be indicated to eliminate the possibility of a thymoma, which is present in about 15% of patients with Myasthenia Gravis. EMG may be performed as a confirmatory test as well. The classic EMG finding in Myasthenia Gravis is the electrodecremental response to repetitive stimulation. An MRI of the brain would not be needed.

565. Answer: D

The correct "incorrect" answer is seizures, if they develop, usually begin between 12-15 months of age. This patient most likely has Sturge-Weber syndrome since the port-wine nevus involves the trigeminal nerve and is therefore at risk for neuro-ocular abnormalities. Many patients have facial port-wine nevi without eye or brain abnormalities. CNS involvement is variable and includes seizures, paresis, mental deficiency or normal intelligence (39%). Seizures (56% chance) most commonly develop between 2 and 7 months of age and may be asymmetric. Conventional anticonvulsant treatment is of limited value. The cause is unknown and sporadic.

566. Answer: E

The correct answer is subependymal nodular calcifications on CT scan. This patient has seizures and adenoma sebaceum (facial skin hamartomas) which suggests tuberous sclerosis. The pathognomonic finding is subependymal nodular calcifications on CT scan. Sometimes widened gyri or tubers and brain tumors can be seen. Two loci have been identified (9q34 and 16p13) and inheritance is autosomal dominant with >85% representing new mutations. Typical features include facial angiofibromas or subungual fibromas, hypomelanotic macules (ash leaf lesions), shagreen patch (rough, orange-peel lesion usually in lumbosacral region, gingival fibromas, retinal hamartomas, subependymal calcifications/nodules or cortical tubers, and renal angiomyolipomas. Rhabdomyomas of the heart may also occur. Ninety-three percent of patients have seizures while 62% have mental deficiency. The variety of symptoms is variable ranging from asymptomatic except for skin lesions to severe mental retardation. Treatment consists of anticonvulsant therapy and surgical intervention for tubers causing intracranial obstruction or tumors.

567. Answer: C

The correct answer is astrocytoma. Cerebellar astrocytoma is the most common posterior fossa tumor in childhood. They tend to be cystic but may have no cystic cavitation. The tumor causes increased intracranial pressure by blocking the fourth ventricle. Tumors involving the cerebellar hemisphere cause ipsilateral extremity ataxia whereas those involving the vermis (midline) cause gait/truncal ataxia. Treatment is surgical resection with a 90% 5-year survival rate. Radiation therapy is reserved for those patients with high-grade tumors.

568. Answer: D

The answer is immediate consultation with ENT. This patient has fever, sore throat, dysphagia, trismus, asymmetric tonsillar swelling, and deviation of the uvula. These are all symptoms of peritonsillar abscess, which requires surgical drainage in addition to antibiotics.

569. Answer: A

The correct answer is 24 hours after his IM injection. Note, that it doesn't make any difference if he receives IM or oral antibiotics on his return to school. Either requires 24 hours after the initial dose of antibiotics.

570. Answer: A

The correct answer is *Arcanobacterium haemolyticum*. This organism has been described for over 10 years as an increasingly common cause of pharyngitis in young adults and adolescents. The organism can only be cultivated on blood-enriched media—which means it is rarely looked for in standard labs. Treatment is with erythromycin or penicillin. No long-term adverse effects are known for non-treatment of this organism which usually resolves without specific therapy. It does not cause Rheumatic fever or glomerulonephritis.

571. Answer: C

The correct answer is *Mycobacterium avium-intracellulare*. This is commonly seen in preschool children. It usually results from coming in contact with the organism in the environment—like playing outside in the dirt. The cure is total excision. MRSA would be a possibility but—amazingly in community acquired MRSA infections; "regular" antibiotics seem to work for these skin infections. You would expect some improvement at least initially. *Mycobacterium marinum* would be seen if he had exposure to a fish tank and usually lymphadenopathy occurs along areas of the water exposure—for example along a forearm that is frequently being dipped into a fish tank. Lymphoma and leukemia are much less likely as a cause of a single lymph node. Look for more signs and symptoms in the history to help you think of these 2 entities.

572. Answer: B

The correct "incorrect" answer is tympanometry can measure hearing sensitivity. It is really only good for determining the architecture and function of the tympanic membrane. Thus a flat line or "low amplitude" tympanogram is associated with middle ear fluid or an obstructed tympanostomy tube. You can have a normal tympanogram and have significant sensorineural hearing loss; or you can have an abnormal tympanogram and having perfectly normal hearing. They may not be related. Thus, tympanometry is NOT a good measure of hearing sensitivity.

573. Answer: D

The correct answer is school age children. This age group can cooperate with the commands. This test tests each ear independently and can differentiate between sensorineural and conductive hearing loss. Remember sitting in that room with all of the other kids and putting on the headphones—and listening to that "bell" or "bing" sound? Infants less than 6 months of age and newborns are screened first usually with "behavioral observational audiometry". If the screen is positive then they go on to brainstem-evoked auditory potential—auditory brainstem response (ABR). For 6-month-olds to 2 years—you can use visual reinforcement audiometry—this tests for bilateral hearing loss so that you can intervene to prevent language problems from developing.

574. Answer: D

The correct answer is administration of aminoglycoside while in the neonatal intensive care unit. Of the items listed, this is the only one that causes a sensorineural hearing loss—the other cause a conductive hearing loss. Other causes of sensorineural hearing loss include the loop diuretics (furosemide and ethacrynic acid) and salicylate toxicity. Viral infections can sometimes cause acute deafness also.

575. Answer: A

The correct answer is perilymph fistula. This occurs with an abnormal tract develops between the inner and middle ear. This results in loss of perilymph. The patients usually have vertigo and ataxia with hearing loss. Ménière's Disease is very, very rare in kids. It will usually present with tinnitus.

576. Answer: C

The correct answer is foreign body. Most likely little Bridget has a piece of corn or something yummy stuck up in there. The key here is the painful movement of the pinna without evidence of infection—there is no redness or swelling of the pinna. Otitis externa is likely here but the foreign body is the culprit.

577. Answer: E

The correct answer is cocaine abuse. The perforated nasal septum and the chronic congestion in a teenager or young adult should make you think of cocaine or other inhaled substances. You need to address this before you move on to the more "mundane" causes. The lack of eosinophils helps you to move seasonal allergic rhinitis out of the picture.

578. Answer: C

The correct answer is cold-induced cold abscesses (or popsicle panniculitis). No treatment is necessary and these will clear over the next few weeks. They do not usually leave any type of scarring or long-term effects.

579. Answer: A

The correct answer is to ask the mother to bring the baby for examination. Dacryostenosis, or congenital nasolacrimal duct obstruction, occurs in approximately 6% of newborns. It occurs when the epithelial cells lining the nasolacrimal gland fail to canalize. Signs include overflow of tears and production of mucinous material from the lacrimal sac. Infection or inflammation may occur in the nasolacrimal sac or surrounding tissues. Rarely, a periorbital cellulitis occurs. Traditional treatment includes gentle massage and eye washing. 96% resolve in the first year of life. Ophthalmologic referral for probing is indicated in cases that do not resolve in the first year. The differential diagnosis for excessive tearing includes infantile glaucoma, corneal abrasion, and the presence of a foreign body. For this reason, an exam is indicated in any infant with the complaint of excessive tearing.

580. Answer: C

The correct answer is refer for immediate evaluation by an ophthalmologist. 30% of infants with glaucoma demonstrate all components of the classic triad of infantile glaucoma, which includes excessive tearing, photophobia, and blepharospasm. Other signs and symptoms include corneal edema, corneal and ocular enlargement, conjunctival injection, and visual impairment. Any infant suspected of having a nasolacrimal duct obstruction should be evaluated for signs and symptoms of glaucoma. Surgery to relieve intraocular pressure is immediately indicated once the diagnosis of glaucoma is made. Disorders and conditions associated with infantile glaucoma include galactosemia, trauma, intraocular hemorrhage, ocular inflammatory disease, Sturge-Weber syndrome, Marfan's syndrome, von Recklinghausen disease, Lowe syndrome, congenital rubella, and juvenile xanthogranuloma among others. Immediate ophthalmologic referral is indicated when the diagnosis is suspected.

581. Answer: A

The correct answer is *Bacillus cereus*. Let's "be serious" for a moment (Ok, bad ID Joke.) This is an obvious emergency and this organism is a bad one. It is associated with penetrating injury to the eyeball. Remember also that it causes food poisoning particularly the "Chinese rice-bowl" variety. *Acanthamoeba* is associated with contact lenses and solutions—so think about that if they give you a patient with that type of scenario. *Staphylococcus epidermidis*—think about after ocular surgery—particularly cataract extraction or lens implantation. It can also occur after trauma but *B. cereus* is one of the few that will give you a ring abscess: Pseudomonas and Proteus are about the only other two agents that will do that too. *Bartonella henselae*—no kitties around in the history and usually you'll get a conjunctivitis picture NOT this nasty scenario. So just remember penetrating eye injury with ring abscess formation in the cornea: *B. cereus*!

582. Answer: E

The correct "incorrect" answer is exotropia is more common than esotropia. The other statements listed are true. Esotropia is the most common form of strabismus in childhood. Esotropia is defined as when the child is "cross-eyed". Exotropia is defined when the child is "wall-eyed". Deviation upward is "hypertropia" and deviation downward is "hypotropia".

583. Answer: E

The correct answer is the majority of children with significant refractory errors have no complaints whatsoever. This is why screening should occur in children after the 2nd year of life. Myopia is nearsightedness and is rare in early term infants—it is more common in preterm infants and others with retinopathy of prematurity. Hyperopia usually does NOT require spectacle correction if mild. Most adults are hyperopic. Contact lenses can be quite useful in childhood especially for conditions such as the aphakic child.

584. Answer: D

The correct answer is craniopharyngioma. Chiasmal lesions interrupt the central fibers that mediate temporal vision—therefore a pituitary tumor or craniopharyngioma results in loss of visual fields in the bitemporal regions. If the lesion was posterior to the chiasm—such as loss of visual cortex in one occipital lobe—a complete loss of visual perception in one field would result.

585. Answer: A

The correct answer is left sympathetic chain. The symptoms are consistent with sympathetic denervation of her left eye—the "Horner" pupil. Most commonly pulmonary neoplasms of the superior sulcus will produce this lesion. Usually it is associated with ipsilateral ptosis and anhidrosis. Pupillary light responses should be normal, as should the response to agents that dilate and constrict the pupil. However, since the sympathetic chain is not working, cocaine cannot cause local release of sympathomimetic substances and is a poor dilator.

586. Answer: D

The correct answer is congenital glaucoma. Now me, personally—I would have jumped right at that stupid congenital cataracts answer—but, cataracts do not cause blepharospasm and enlarged corneas. What the heck is that stupid word epiphora?? That means excessive tearing.

587. Answer: D

The correct answer is retinopathy of prematurity. This is also known as retrolental fibroplasia. This is a major concern with HYPEROXEMIA. Generally, we like to keep the PaO2 below 100 mm Hg because of this.

588. Answer: E

The correct answer is they are always abnormal. They actually are associated with Down's syndrome babies and are tiny white dots that form a ring in the mid-zone of the iris. However, they can occur in up to 25% of "normal" kids especially those with blue eyes.

589. Answer: E

The answer is no intervention--the problem will resolve itself with time. Internal tibial torsion is the most common cause of intoeing in children 2 years of age and younger. It may be associated with metatarsus adductus. This condition usually resolves without intervention. Rarely, the torsion persists in the older child and requires surgical intervention. Other causes of intoeing include internal femoral torsion, metatarsus adductus, and clubfoot. Metatarsus adductus occurs when the forefoot is adducted. This adduction may be flexible or rigid. This disorder may be identified by following a line that bisects the base of the hindfoot forward to the toes. In the normal foot, this line should pass between the second and third toes. If it passes lateral to this, there is metatarsus adductus. Clubfoot occurs as the result of dislocation of the talonavicular joint. Examination of the clubfoot reveals hindfoot equinus, hindfoot and midfoot varus, and forefoot adduction. Internal femoral rotation is demonstrated by the entire lower leg being inwardly rotated while walking.

590. Answer: E

The answer is no intervention--the problem will resolve itself. The most common cause of intoeing in a child greater than 2 years of age is internal femoral torsion. In the prone position, there is 80-90 degrees of internal rotation of the hip. External rotation is limited to less than 10 degrees. Generalized ligamentous laxity may be present. Radiographic evaluation is not necessary. Generally, the problem self corrects and no intervention is necessary. If the deformity persists beyond 10 years of age, surgical intervention may be necessary.

591. Answer: A

The answer is Legg-Calve-Perthes disease or avascular necrosis of the femoral head. Legg-Calve-Perthes disease, or avascular necrosis of the capital femoral epiphysis occurs after an interruption of blood flow to the capital femoral head. It is more likely to affect males than females, occurs between 2 and 12 years of age, and may be bilateral (20%). Children typically present with intermittent thigh pain and limp. An antalgic gait, muscle spasm, and restriction of abduction and internal rotation may occur. Short stature may also be present. Radiographic evaluation may demonstrate any of five stages of the disease including cessation of epiphyseal growth, subchondral fracture, resorption, reossification, or healed, residual stage. Treatment options range from careful observation to surgical intervention depending on the age of the child and the severity of the changes in the femoral head. Children with this disorder should be followed closely by an orthopedic surgeon.

592. Answer: E

The correct answer is X-ray of the elbow. This child likely has a radial head subluxation, or nurse maid's elbow. The point tenderness, in addition to the secondary trauma make it difficult to rule out a fracture. When a fracture is possible, reduction should not be attempted until radiographic evidence has ruled out a fracture. Positioning for the radiograph may result in reduction. You'll notice this question is similar to another one in the ortho section—but note the choices..the choice of "E" is the least invasive. Sometimes you have to look for the "best" answer—even though it may not be what you are really looking for.

593. Answer: C

The correct answer is physical exam only. This patient has Osgood-Schlatter disease which is the most common apophysitis. It is caused by repeated microtrauma to the apophyseal cartilage at the site of tendon insertion. Physical findings include tenderness over the tibial tubercles which can also be elicited by knee extension against resistance or by passive knee flexion. X-rays are only indicated to rule out other causes of tender bone swelling and are probably not needed for bilateral involvement. If the patient had only one side involved, x-rays would be necessary to rule out other causes including osteogenic sarcoma. Treatment includes rest, ice, and proper stretching.

594. Answer: A

The correct answer is increased genu valgum in a 3-year-old. The normal physiologic development of the tibiofemoral angle progresses as follow:

Birth--2 years: varus (bowing) of the knees
2—4 years: valgus (knock-knee) posture
4—7 years: levels off to 4-7 degrees valgus in males and 5-9 degrees in females

595. Answer: B

The correct answer is supinate the forearm and then flex the elbow. This patient has subluxation of the radial head or nursemaid's elbow that is reduced by the maneuver described. It occurs when longitudinal traction is applied while the elbow is extended resulting in the annular ligament becoming partially entrapped in the radiohumeral joint. The child will usually hold the forearm in a pronated position against the body with the elbow slightly bent and will refuse to use the arm. Pain is usually only elicited with movement of the elbow. X-rays are usually not necessary. With reductions as described above, a "click" will be felt along the lateral aspect of the elbow. A child has increased risk for subluxation after the first episode. You'll notice this question is similar to another one in the ortho section—but note the choices..the choice of "B" is the least invasive as the answer was for the one that asked you to get an x-ray. Sometimes you have to look for the "best" answer—even though it may not be what you are really looking for.

596. Answer: A

The answer is CBC. This patient has the typical symptoms of growing pains including chronic, recurrent, nighttime leg pain that is relieved with simple measures. Episodes usually occur several times per week, and the pain is bilateral (most often generalized along the anterolateral leg or calf muscles). The pain is resolved by the next day and there is no limp. Physical exam is normal. Although growing pains are benign and usually resolve within months-2 years, leukemia should be considered and ruled out with a CBC. Radiographs are normal and should only be obtained if the history is atypical or unclear. Further evaluation is necessary with atypical history such as limp, pain during the day, well-located or unilateral pain, or joint swelling. Stretching and application of a heating pad may help with growing pains.

597. Answer: B

The correct answer is 11 years for girls, 11.5 years for boys. The range for girls is from 8 to 13 years and for boys it is 9.5 to 13.5 years. Adolescence is considered from ages 10 to 21 years.

598. Answer: C

The correct answer is 25%. Another of those exciting facts you just need to burn in your mind for the ABP!

599. Answer: D

The correct answer is for girls, Tanner stage 2-3; for boys Tanner stage 4. Note, (as usually is the case), boys are delayed compared to girls. Girls will reach their final height at a mean age of 16 and boys generally will reach their final height at a mean age of 18.

600. Answer: A

The correct answer is the weight of the heart doubles. Generally most organs of the body will increase in size—except the brain (sorry). Lean body mass in boys actually INCREASES to 90% from 80% and mean body fat in boys Increases from 4.3% to 11.2%. Girls also see an INCREASE in body fat from 15.7% to 26.7%. So adolescence really does stink!—Your brain doesn't grow and your body fat increases markedly!

601. Answer: D

The correct answer is 12 years for cigarettes and 12.6 years for alcohol! Remember these are MEAN numbers, which means that many kids start younger than that!

602. Answer: A

The correct answer is 78% boys and 63% of girls have had sex before their 20th birthday.

603. Answer: A

The correct answer is 92% for African-American boys and 77% for African-American girls. Hispanic children's rates are 79% for boys and 57% for girls. Rates for Caucasian boys and girls are78% and 63% respectively.

604. Answer: B

The correct answer is discuss her recent history briefly with the parents and then ask them to wait in the waiting room while you take a complete history and examine the patient. Note she is at an age where she should be seen without her parents. You really don't have a clue if this could be gonorrhea or something else (ok, it is most likely Mono or less likely *Streptococcus pyogenes*)—but still the ABP wants you to know that the adolescent should be treated as an adult in this situation. You should not give the parents a choice and you really cannot put the child on the spot—"You want your parents to stay or go?" What is the 'smart' child going to say? "Oh no, they can stay it is no big deal." This will prevent you from getting to the true adolescent issues that need to be addressed and she may have a question that she won't ask in front of the parents. Today you will have a staff person assist you in the examination room if you are the opposite sex—and many make it a practice to do this for ALL patients regardless of gender—Remember the idyllic times only occur in Reruns!

605. Answer: D

The correct answer is depression—pretty obvious of those choices, I hope? The problem with adolescent depression is frequently it is unrecognized. Usually it will present as a weird constellation of symptoms from eating problems, sleeping problems, dysphoric mood, low self-esteem, and somatic complaints.

606. Answer: A

The correct answer is depression. She has all of the "classic" adolescent signs of depression that occur in teenagers: eating problems, sleep disturbance, dysphoric mood, low self-esteem, and somatic complaints. She has no physical findings to support hypo- or hyperthyroidism and she is very unlikely to have a "vitamin deficiency".

607. Answer: C

The correct answer is MMR and offer her meningococcal vaccine. She needs a 2nd MMR and somehow missed receiving it during her 12 year-old check up. She is not due for a Td for another 4 years unless she has a tetanus-prone injury. Meningococcal vaccine should be offered to all college freshmen—particularly those who will be living in dormitories---the vaccine has been shown to be useful in preventing meningococcal disease in this discrete population. She received her varicella vaccine before the age of 13 and therefore only one dose is required. Currently, hepatitis B booster after the 3-dose regimen is not recommended routinely.

608. Answer: A

The correct answer is Papanicolaou smear, RPR, HIV counseling, GC and *Chlamydia* culturing, and empiric treatment of GC and Chlamydia. Note that HSV culturing is not likely to be helpful. If she is asymptomatic you would not treat her even if she had positive cultures and it would not be causing her discharge. Culturing for *Gardnerella* is not cost-effective, is difficult to do, and likely would not yield meaningful results. *Candida* culturing is not going to be helpful. She likely is colonized and so even if you find the organism it doesn't necessarily mean that it is causing the problem. You must determine if she has gonorrhea or *Chlamydia*. Both are treatable diseases and it is important for her to know and for the public health officials in the community to be aware of either of these infections so that partner notification can occur. Also you would empirically treat her at this point, knowing that she may not return for effective therapy.

609. Answer: B

The correct answer is 33.3%. This question asks you to calculate the sensitivity of a new test (LEUKALERT) in a defined patient population. To calculate sensitivity, it is the number of patients with a positive LEUKALERT who have leukemia (true positives) divided by the number of all patients with leukemia in the study (true positives *plus* false negatives). For this case it would be 12 (the number of patients who are LEUKALERT positive and who have leukemia) divided by 12 (those who are LEUKALERT Positive and have leukemia)+ 24 (those with leukemia who had a negative LEUKALERT test).

12/(12+24) = 12/36 = 1/3 = 33.3%

610. Answer: A

The correct answer is 12.5%. Positive predictive value is obtained by taking True positives divided by (true positives + false positives). In this case 25/(25+175) = 12.5%

611. Answer: A

The correct answer is 98.9%. The negative predictive value is True Negatives divided by (false negatives + true negatives). In this case: 890/ (10 +890) = 98.9%.

612. Answer: E

The correct answer is No. The key here is the 95% confidence interval. It crosses over 0. This indicates that the differences between the new treatment and the standard therapy were NOT statistically significant. The numbers can be quite deceiving--even with such a large increase in survival. One possibility is that the study had too few patients to really have any power to show a significant difference between the two groups.

613. Answer: A

The correct answer is 5. Number of people needed to treat to prevent one bad outcome is based on 1 divided by (absolute risk reduction) = 1 divided by (the rate in the placebo group minus the rate in treatment group). In our example: 1/(20/50 – 10/50) = 1/(.4-.2) = 1/(.2) = 5

614. Answer: C

The correct answer is 71.4%. To calculate sensitivity you take True positives divided by (True positives + false negatives). In this case: 25/(25+10) = 71.4%

615. Answer: D

The correct answer is 83.5%. To calculate specificity you take True negatives divided by (True negatives + false positives). In this case: 890/(890 + 175) = 83.5%